# MIDWIFERY MANAGEMENT OF TWIN GESTATIONS

# MIDWIFERY MANAGEMENT OF TWIN GESTATIONS

*An Evidence – Based Approach*

By B. Maria Cranford, CPM MSM

Mountain Home Books

Printed in the United States of America

First Printing, 2015

ISBN 978-0692513644

Mountain Home Books
362 E Ashlyn LN
Draper, UT 84020

www.mountainhomebirth.com/store


Cover Photos Copyright © 2010 by Leilani Rogers, photographer
www.photosbylei.com

# DEDICATION

*To my dear husband and munchkins - the journey has been long and I could
never have done this without each one of you*

*and*

*To the One who gave the beginning inspiration and continues giving precious
guidance day by day*

# ACKNOWLEDGMENTS

Much love and appreciation to Dianne, Courtney, Karen, April and Nicole, for their support and encouragement throughout the long research and writing process

# CONTENTS

## LIST OF TABLES AND FIGURES

# 1 INTRODUCTION

In the United States, where and with whom a woman should deliver her baby is a topic of current, intense deliberation. Across multiple countries including the United States, studies show that outcomes for low-risk, planned home birth with a trained attendant give positive maternal infant health outcomes and allow for "high rates of physiologic birth and low rates of intervention without an increase in adverse outcomes" (Cheyney et al., 2014, p. 17; see also Hutton, Reitsma, & Kaufman, 2009; Lindgren, Radestad, Christensson, & Hildingsson, 2008; Symon, Winter, Inkster, & Donnan, 2009). Although studies have found safety in birth occurring in home and birth center settings, the literature has not found one setting as the "safest birthing place for all women" (Albers & Katz, 1991, p. 215; Likis, 2014). In fact, Likis (2014) called "determining which women are appropriate candidates for home birth" one of the "primary unresolved challenges related to the safety of home birth in the United States" (p. 567).

Furthermore, midwife-led twin birth in home and birth center settings gives rise to even greater disagreement. Currently, "there are no national guidelines in the United States that list conditions for which home birth is not recommended" (Likis, 2014, p. 567). However, the American College of Obstetricians and Gynecologists (ACOG) has issued Committee Opinion Number 476 on Planned Home Birth that, while respecting "the right of women to make a medically informed decision about delivery," specified twin birth as having a greater risk of perinatal death and asserted that twin gestation placed a candidate at too high a risk for home birth, a stance agreed upon by the American Academy of Pediatrics (ACOG Committee on Obstetric Practice, 2011, p. 425; Watterberg & AAP Committee on Fetus and Newborn, 2013).

Yet, as recently as the years spanning 2004-2010, midwives attended the vast majority of births in homes and birth centers and the proportion of multiple births in those settings was consistent throughout the time frame of the study (with multiple births accounting for 1.0% of home births and 0.3% of birth center births compared to 3.5% of hospital births) (MacDorman, Declercq, & Mathews, 2013).

Additionally, Grünebaum et al. (2015), in examining birth certificate data on perinatal risks among planned home births in the United States from the Centers for Disease Control (CDC), showed certified nurse midwives (CNMs) were managing deliveries of twins in hospital (n=2276) and in homes and birth centers (n=101) while demonstrating that other midwives were also facilitating twin births in birth centers and homes (n=256). Indeed, in detailing results of a survey among certified professional midwives (CPMs) about scope of practice, Darragh (2012) reported that one-third of CPMs felt management of twin gestation to be within the purview of their practice. Further, while stating that "the safety net available in an institutional setting is advantageous and may be preferable for" twin gestation, breech presentation and trial of labor after cesarean (TOLAC), Cook, Avery and Frisvold (2014) acknowledged that some "CNMs/CMs [certified nurse midwives/certified midwives] attending home births may have the skill to attend such births" at home (p. 157). Hence, no clear consensus exists on the appropriate birth place for mothers with twin gestation. Additionally, when choosing to deliver twins in home and birth center settings, evidence-based management guidelines are not well defined. Therefore, this book seeks to describe the current climate in regards to twin birth in homes and birth centers, reviewing the literature, both historical and current, of midwife-led care of twin gestation and then to describe the core skill set necessary for midwives to successfully facilitate twin gestation within a home and birth center setting.

# 2 EXAMINING THE LITERATURE ON MIDWIFERY CARE OF TWIN GESTATION

When examining midwifery-led care of twin gestation, the limited literature on the topic can be divided into historical and contemporary care of twins by midwives. Documented care of twins by midwives during the 20th century can be found within reports and studies that chronicle individual midwives' practices as well as limited outcome data contained within analysis on planned home births. When it can be found, information on more contemporary care of twins by midwives focuses on morbidity and mortality outcomes, both within overall planned home and birth center data analysis and through specifically delineated outcomes associated with midwifery-led twin care.

## Historical Midwifery Care of Twins

Historically, there is evidence of the management of twins in the home setting. For example, in 1996, Allison analyzed data on the Nottingham district midwives in England from the years 1949 to 1972. While the data is quite dated, within this district the home birth rate was over 50% as late as 1963. From 1956-1967, over 36,000 home births occurred and detailed records were kept on multiple births taking place within the district (Allison, 1996, p. xix).

During this window of time, 189 sets of twins and one set of triplets were delivered at home, some being diagnosed prior to delivery and others diagnosed after labor had begun (Allison, 1996). From the records, 170 twin sets and a set of triplets were delivered (or attended immediately after the birth) by a district midwife with no record of a doctor in attendance (Allison, 1996). Twenty of the twin sets have more information available through the attending midwives' personal registers. While too small a data set from which to draw conclusions, these twin births give unique insight into the historical facilitation of twin home birth by midwives.

Among theses births are factors that would seemingly place the birth outside the sphere of a planned home birth and Allison (1996) suggests a contemporary, reasonable course of action would be to insure delivery in the hospital: primigravida (n=2), grand-multiparae (n=3), advanced maternal age (n=2), 42+ weeks gestational age (n=2), no prenatal care and premature 34 weeks gestational age (n=1). Yet, escalation of care seemed to happen appropriately, as 19 of the 40 babies were born weighing less than 5lb 8oz, and only 4 of those newborns were recognized to need specialized care and transferred to the hospital, and two other babies were transferred to the hospital for unknown reasons (Allison, 1996). Allison (1996) puts forward that clinical "judgment and selection" were made by the midwives as to which babies would have an enhanced chance of survival with the support provided by a hospital (p. 98). Also, within this subset of district babies, the only deaths were two stillbirths within a single set of twins (Allison, 1996). In this one case, the mother had been referred for care with hypertension early in pregnancy and then returned to the care of the midwife. "The consultant obstetrician performed a surgical induction at home; both twins were stillborn, the second was hydrocephalic" (Allison, 1996, p. 98). Although no more information is available in regards to this birth, since the medical induction occurred at home, the author postulates that the intrauterine fetal death of both twins may have been already diagnosed (Allison, 1996).

Additionally, another study documents twins placed within a midwife's scope of practice as well as showing twin birth being part of the "lower risk" category of planned home and birth center births. In analyzing midwifery client selection in the Netherlands between 1969 and 1983, van Alten, Eskes and Treffers (1989) gathered data from within a single practice of midwives who were facilitating births in a freestanding "maternity home" birthing center and in local homes within their "catchment area" of 40,000 inhabitants. Choice of birth site was made by the pregnant woman, with a high proportion of the births taking place at the maternity home, located in the center of the catchment area. Complications were transferred both prenatally and intrapartum to local physicians and hospitals. During the time frame, 7980 women consecutively booked with the midwives, including 75 sets of twins. Although the specific outcomes of the twins are not delineated in the study, it is interesting to note that (1) a twin gestation did not automatically transfer clients out of midwifery care, (2) twin gestation was considered an "uncomplicated pregnancy," and (3) that the choice remained for birth at the client's home or the "maternity home" (van Alten, Eskes, & Treffers, 1989, p. 657). The study found that practicing midwives are able to self-select clients based on their own criteria of "high risk" and achieve safe outcomes for birth in homes and birth centers (van Alten et al., 1989).

## Contemporary Twin Outcomes

More recent research documents the continued midwifery-led management of twin gestation in home and birth center settings, but the literature remains scarce in regards to the specificities of outcomes and characteristics of twin gestation. The current literature on twin gestation in the home and birth center setting uses one of three overarching approaches in the reporting of twin outcomes: 1) the study includes twins as part of an overall analysis of home and birth center birth data wherein the twin subset is not specifically delineated in the study analysis; 2) the study excludes twin sets from the data altogether and/or records the transfer of care for twin gestation prior to labor; or 3) the study reports some outcomes associated specifically with twin gestation (Cheng, Snowden, King, & Caughey, 2013).

However, the dearth of robust literature that exists on morbidity and mortality for twin gestation associated with midwifery–led care in home and birth center settings remains a large contributing factor to the lack of consensus on delivery site for twin gestation and associated management thereof. In reviewing over 150 home and birth center articles for twin-specific outcomes, including all articles contained in Vedam's (2013) *Home birth: An annotated guide to the literature* and other, more current, articles found using similar criteria as Vedam's review, country of origin for the study became an important factor to consider, as outcomes for low-resource countries may not be completely applicable to high-resource countries such the United States. In addition, other high-resource countries, such as the United Kingdom, Canada, New Zealand and the Netherlands have more integrated home and birth center services within their countries' maternity care system. The United States lacks such integration, making extrapolating their outcomes for pertinence in the United States somewhat difficult. Regardless, the following sections review those articles including data on midwife-led twin birth in homes and birth centers in high-resource countries.

**Twin (as part of low-risk group) outcomes.** A strong example of the first approach can be found in a meta-analysis by Olsen (1997). In this meta-analysis, one of the included studies had twins (sample size for twin subset not defined) in their data set (Olsen, 1997). The meta-analysis itself showed decreased morbidity without poor secondary outcomes in the home birth group with data not sufficient for mortality statistics, but no information specific to the twins was reported.

In an early evaluation of home and birth center births attended by study-defined "experienced," non-certified nurse midwives, Mehl et al. (1980) included one set of twins in their data set for both the experienced midwives and the matched physician cohort. While outcomes for the twin set were not delineated, the study showed major differences in management style between the physicians and midwives with better outcomes and lower intervention rates favoring the experienced midwives when compared to the physicians.

Furthermore, a study of 11,788 planned home births with CNMs stated 4% of participating practices in the study included twin and breech birth as part of their scope of practice (Anderson & Murphy, 1995). All of the midwives who included twin and breech birth in their scope of practice had been in home birth practice for five years or more. This particular study demonstrated planned home birth with a qualified provider is a safe alternative for healthy "lower risk" women (Anderson & Murphy, 1995).

**Exclusion of twins from outcome data.** Another study analyzing perinatal and maternal outcomes in planned home births among women at "higher risk" of complications specifically excluded multiple gestation from their data set (Li et al., 2015). Further, Cox et al. (2013) analyzed home births outcomes during a 25 year period among the Amish in southeastern Pennsylvania, with the twin gestations (n=2) in the data set transferring care prenatally.

**Delineated twin outcomes.** In addition to the above, a number of articles were found specifically listing outcome information of twin home and birth center births within the discussion section of their study data. Janssen et al. (2002) studied outcomes of planned home births after the regulation of midwifery in British Columbia. Included in the study were three sets of twins, two of which were undiagnosed prior to delivery. The diagnosed twin set delivered in the hospital. Of the two sets of twins born at home, no baby was breech presentation and APGAR scores for all twin babies were seven or more at one minute and eight or more at five minutes, similar to the APGAR scores for the total hospital cohort (Janssen et al., 2002). Another study reported on 49 twin gestations among 1462 pregnancies managed by independent midwives in the United Kingdom (Symon, Winter, Inkster, & Donnan, 2009). Six deaths occurred to planned home birth twins: 2 had lethal anomalies; 1 was <34 weeks gestation and vaginal breech; 2 were vaginal breech second twins; and 1 was an intrapartum transfer with an operative breech. No discussion is made in the article about the size of the vaginal breech second twins relative to the first twin, nor the preterm nature of the <34 gestational age twin.

Further, while Johnson and Daviss (2005) removed the twin home birth and breech subsets from their home birth data for analysis of outcomes, they reported the mortality statistics for these subsets within their outcome discussion. Although reporting a 2.5% mortality rate for singleton breeches, the data revealed no deaths in the 13 sets of twins with CPM management in the home birth setting (Johnson & Daviss, 2005). Another study analyzed perinatal death in Australia with planned home birth (Bastian, Keirse, & Lancaster, 1998). Although the total number of twin births is not given in the article, the authors do attribute two of the 23 intrapartum asphyxial deaths to second twins. As pointed out by Vedam (2011), the midwives whose data were included in the study were unregistered, and many had limited training, scant experience and little, if any, access to resuscitation equipment. Such births "without qualified attendants are not consistent with definitions of planned home birth in most countries" (Vedam, 2011, p. 11). Kennare, Kierse, Tucker and Chan (2010) also investigated 1141 planned home births in South Australia from 1991-2006. Of the five sets of twins that planned to deliver at home, five infants were born at home with the second twin in the third set dying of intrapartum asphyxia due to the "mother refusing a hospital birth and a difficult transfer in labor" (Anderson & Stone, 2013, p. 66). The other two sets of twins were born in the hospital (Kennare et al., 2010).

Moreover, a recent analysis of the Midwives Alliance of North America Statistics Project for the years 2004-2009 revealed data on 60 sets of twins (Cheyney et al., 2014). Although absolute numbers show one intrapartum death in the 120 babies born within the twin subset, statistical analysis showed "no evidence of increased risk of death among multiple births" at home (Cheyney et al., 2014, pp. 23, 24). However, in their discussion, the authors do include multiple gestations within the group of "women who are at higher risk for adverse outcomes" (Cheyney et al., 2014, p. 25). The authors conclude their study by stating that:

Low-risk women in this sample experienced high rates of normal physiologic birth and very low rates of operative birth and interventions, with no concomitant increase in adverse events. Conclusions are less clear for higher-risk women. Given the low absolute number of events and the lack of a matched comparison group, we were unable to discern whether poorer outcomes among higher-risk women were associated with place of birth or related to risks inherent to their conditions (Cheyney et al., 2014, p. 26).

Finally, in the only study found analyzing twin-specific outcomes in midwife-attended home birth, Mehl-Madrona and Madrona (1997) found a statistically significant increase in perinatal mortality when twin, breech and post-dates data were included together in the sample.

In their discussion and conclusion, they make the case for higher risk in these clients and a need for hospital delivery with twins, breeches and postdates births. However, in analyzing the actual charted data, if just the postdates' births are removed (leaving the twin and breech birth in the data set), the difference in perinatal mortality is once again non-significant (Mehl-Madrona & Madrona, 1997, p. 95). Wagner (1998) pointed out this fact in a letter to the editor of the journal the following year, stating, "that while including post-date cases significantly increases the perinatal mortality rate of planned home birth, including twin and breech birth does not significantly increase the perinatal mortality rate of planned home birth" (p. 121). In their response beginning on the same page, the study's authors revealed that their conclusions were drawn from the fact that, although twin and breech birth did not meet "statistical significance," it was of borderline significance (Madrona & Mehl-Madrona, 1998). The most interesting part of the whole study is the following quote from the authors' response letter to the editor:

We would add that were we personally to have a breech baby or twins, *we would probably want them to be born at home* (emphasis added). Yet, standard of care for a society must be based on what is safest for mothers and babies. At this time, it is recognized that breeches and twins necessitate a greater skill in assessing their risk and assisting at their deliveries and, therefore, *more studies should be done to determine what skill is necessary for their safest outcomes* (emphasis added) (Madrona & Mehl-Madrona, 1998, p. 122).

Unfortunately, in the 17 years since the above statement, additional studies have not been done to determine what exact skill set is necessary to successfully facilitate twin birth in home and birth center settings. Until such studies are done, a definitive answer on what setting is best for twin birth will not be available. However, historical and current literature demonstrates that twin gestation continues to take place in home and birth center settings under the management of midwifery-led models of care (Cook, Avery, & Frisvold, 2014; MacDorman, Declercq, & Mathews, 2013). Given this continued prevalence, evidence-based guidelines for the management of twin births must be developed. The second portion of this book is dedicated to delineating such guidelines, thus allowing a midwife to evaluate skill sets necessary for the successful management and inclusion of twins in her professional scope of practice.

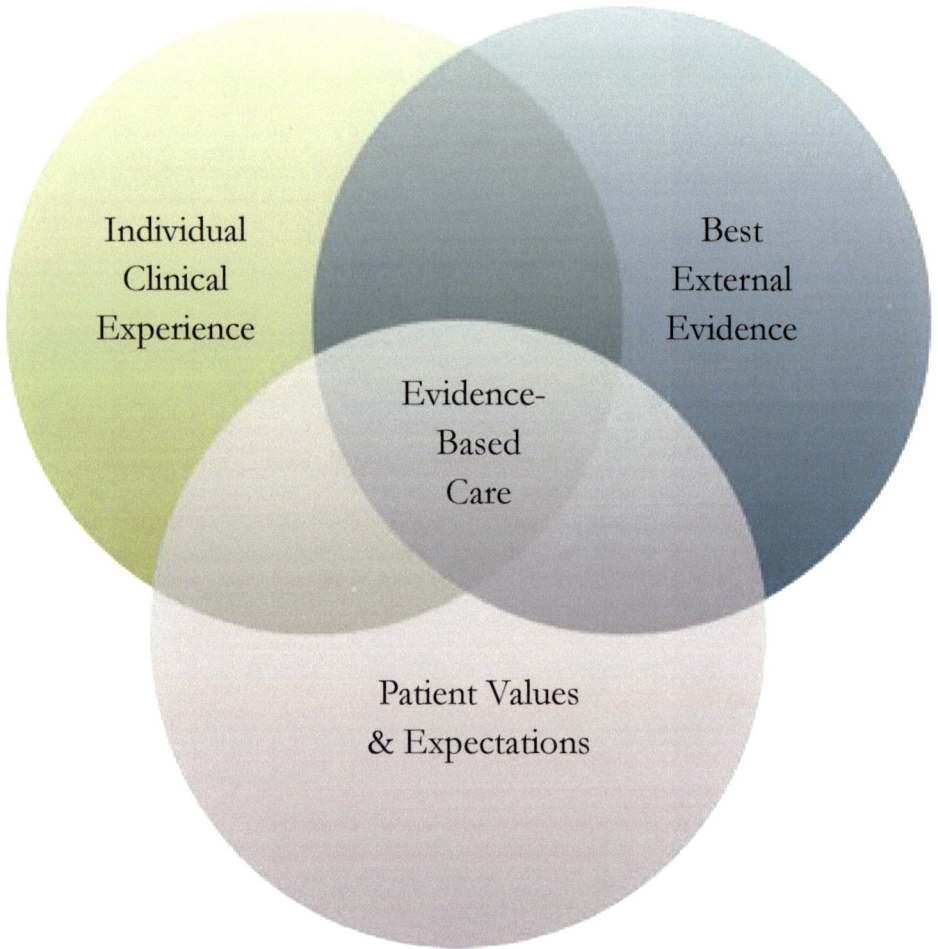

Figure 1. The Evidence-Based Care Triad. Adapted from Sackett, D.L., Rosenberg, W. M.C., Gray, J.A.M., Haynes R.B. and Richardson, W.S. (1996.) Evidenced based medicine: what it is and what it isn't. *BMJ, 312,* 71-72.

# 3 EVIDENCED-BASED MANAGEMENT OF TWIN GESTATION

Evidence-based practice is most appropriately described as a triad of values/ideals working together to formulate the best possible "decisions about the care of the individual patient" (Sackett, 1996, p. 71). These ideals include (1) the provider's clinical expertise, (2) the best research evidence and (3) the patient's values and preferences (Sackett, 1996). The guidelines found within this text seek to inform the second of those three ideals, and, when used within the Midwives Model of Care™ structure, will allow for true evidence-based practice (see Figure 1).

Throughout the childbearing year, midwives strive to provide "individualized education, counseling, and prenatal care, [and] continuous hands-on assistance" in a shared decision-making, "collaborative process that engages the midwife and client in ongoing verbal and written communication about treatment options, … culminat[ing] with informed consent, which can be revisited over time" (Midwifery Task Force, 2008, North American Registry of Midwives, 2014).

However, evidence-based midwifery management of twin gestation is difficult to describe. Starting with the intent to evaluate the current physiologic, midwifery-based evidence, PUBMED was searched for literature informing the various aspects of twin gestation management, limiting the search to current research (last 5-10 years). The dearth of current evidence for twin management from a midwifery background is astounding, with the PUBMED search returning few, if any, peer-reviewed studies in the management areas investigated. This finding was especially true in the area of intrapartum management, where the few articles found were simple descriptions of personal protocols and thoughts by physicians who are open to, and include, vaginal births of twins within their scope of practice (informed by some evidence), or guidelines recommended by professional organizations where evidence is poor for certain guidelines, but the recommendations are made for other reasons (Barrett & Bocking, 2000; Cruikshank, 2007).

Given the scanty results from the initial search for literature, the scope of the search was expanded in both PUBMED and Google Scholar to include backtracking of references in the studies found through the initial search, inclusion of studies from medically-based models of twin management, references used in various midwifery and obstetric textbooks and, then, articles and studies which used the previous studies found as citations. A topics list was generated from the initial studies and texts examined and then expanded based on the further research found regarding twin gestation management. The available evidence is arranged by these topics.

These guidelines are presented in three sections according to progression of the childbearing year: 1) Prenatal Management; 2) Intrapartum Management; and 3) Postpartum Management. Each section presents an overview of normal maternal care through the lens of twin gestation and then reviews complications specific to twin gestation within each period. The book concludes with a review of the importance of professional relationships and standards of practice as well as a discussion about the need for more robust research to inform clinical decisions within a physiologic model of twin gestation and delivery.

# 4 PRENATAL MANAGEMENT OF TWIN GESTATION

Twins are the most common form of multiple gestation in the United States (Leveno & Alexander, 2013). Historically, the twinning rate for the population has been 1 in 80, but the incidence of multifetal gestation has increased 65% in the case of twin pregnancy and 400% where higher-order multiples are concerned (Gabbe, Niebyl, & Simpson, 2007). Much of this increase is due to the various assisted reproduction technologies (ART) available, including fertility drugs such as clomiphene citrate (Clomid) and in-vitro fertilization (Leveno & Alexander, 2013). Surprisingly, unlike the increased risks accompanying singleton pregnancies conceived though ART, risks associated with multiple pregnancies achieved via ART carry only normal risk factors accompanying such pregnancies and, in fact, perinatal mortality seems to be reduced in ART twin pregnancies when compared with spontaneously conceived twin pregnancies (Allen, Wilson, Cheung, Genetics Committee of the Society of Obstetricians & Gynaecologists of Canada, & Reproductive Endocrinology Infertility Committee of the Society of Obstetricians Gynaecologists of Canada, 2006).

## Zygosity and Chorionicity

In discussing twin gestation, the pregnancies can be divided two ways. First, twins can be divided by their zygote formation.

**Monozygotic.** Monozygotic twin gestations are also called "identical twins." Both fetuses came from the same egg and sperm and the fertilized ovum then splits in two. These fetuses share almost the same DNA (less genetic mutations after the split) although they can be of different sizes and personalities. The rate of monozygotic twinning is constant at 1 in 250 (Leveno & Alexander, 2013).

**Dizygotic.** Dizygotic twin gestations are referred to as "fraternal twins." The mother released two separate eggs that were then separately fertilized by two sperm. Fetuses share the same amount of DNA as any two normal siblings. Half of dizygotic twins will be male-female pairs, a quarter will be male-male and a quarter will be female-female. Several factors influence dizygotic twinning including: race (higher with African American women, moderate with white women, and low among Asian women), if the mother herself was a twin, maternal age since hormonal stimulation peaks at age 37, higher parity up to 7, higher incidence with taller and heavier women (hypothesized as being due to greater nutrition) and infertility therapy (Leveno & Alexander, 2013).

Second, twins can also be categorized based on the division of their amnion and chorion. Dizygotic twins will always have two amnion/chorion sacs, one set around each fetus though the placentas may be separate or fused. Monozygotic twins will have one of the three variations of amnion/chorion, depending on the timing of the zygote division (Leveno & Alexander, 2013).

**Dichorionic/diamniotic.** If the zygote divides at days 0-4 after fertilization, the fetuses will have separate sacs, just as the dizygotic twins.

**Monochorionic/diamniotic.**  When division takes place on days 4-8, the twins will share a chorion but be separated by the amnion.

**Monochorionic/monoamniotic.** Twins in this category float together inside both their shared chorion and amnion. The division for these twins happens on days 8-12. This type of pregnancy occurs in 1% of all twin gestations (Barrett & Bocking, 2000).

## Special Considerations during Twin Gestation

While considered a "variation" of normal pregnancy among many direct-entry midwives, hallmarks of twin gestation can be somewhat different from what a midwife would encounter in a singleton gestation (Lay, 2000; Midwifery Today, 2013; Rooks, 1997; Twin Source, 2013).

Once a twin gestation is diagnosed, the normal prenatal appointment needs to be adjusted to allow for these differences. This section discusses these considerations in normal, routine pregnancy care and how some aspects of care may apply differently in a gestation with two fetuses (see Appendix A for a suggested prenatal visit plan for twins).

**Diagnosis of twin gestation.**  Several signs and symptoms would lead to the suspicion of a multiple gestation. See Box on next page.

**Prenatal fetal surveillance in twin gestation.** Certain tests/ screenings that midwives offer to clients have different parameters for use in multiple gestations. These tests include serum screening, amniocentesis and chorionic villus sampling and ultrasounds. Factors influencing the application of these tests in twin gestation are discussed below.

***Serum screening.***  Typically, serum screening tests such as the quad screen return invalid results in twin pregnancies due to the higher

- uterine size/fundal height larger than expected for gestation, especially in the second trimester or after the 20th week;
- severe nausea and vomiting due to increased amounts of hCG;
- family history of twins;
- recent use of ovulation-inducing drugs;
- abdominal palpation of three or more large parts (fetal poles) and/ or multiple small parts; two or more fetal poles in the uterine fundus, especially if the head seems small for the size of the uterus;
- simultaneous comparison of two fetal heartbeats, although only diagnostic when the rate differs by more than ten beats per minute;
- elevated alpha-fetoprotein results; and,
- fetal movement not detected by 18-20 week fundal height

Signs and Symptoms of Multiple Gestation (Fraser, Cooper, & Myles, 2003; Tharpe, Farley, & Jordan, 2013; Varney, Kriebs, & Gegor, 2004).

levels of hormones naturally involved in the pregnancy and the complex interpretation required of the results (Fraser et al., 2003). However, the maternal serum alpha-fetoprotein is "useful for detection of open neural tube and other defects" (Barrett & Bocking, 2000, p. 7).

*Amniocentesis and chorionic villus sampling.* With the risk of Down's Syndrome and other anomalies higher in dizygotic twins than in singletons (Down's Syndrome risk increases at a maternal age of 32 for dizygotic twins versus 35 for singletons), amniocentesis, done between 15 and 20 weeks of pregnancy, seems to be the medical test of choice (Barrett & Bocking, 2000). Usually done by a maternal-fetal medicine specialist, most physicians prefer to do a "dual needle insertion to prevent cross-contamination between sacs" (Fraser, Cooper, & Myles, 2009, p. 438). One study showed a chorionicity-related difference in the fetal death rate after the procedure: 7.7% for monochorionic twins vs. 1.4% among the controls (Vink, Wapner, & D'Alton, 2012).

Although Barrett and Bocking (2000) state that fetal loss rates are unclear with these two procedures, Fraser et al. (2003) recommend that chorionic villus sampling (CVS) not be recommended due to high fetal loss rates in multiple gestation. There is also no guarantee that, during CVS, samples will be successfully taken from each twin (Sperling & Tabor, 2001). In one review, fetal loss rates were slightly higher in CVS (3-4.5%) than in amniocentesis (2.9-4.18%) for multiple gestations (Vink et al., 2012). The review also discussed fetal defects, such as limb reductions, associated with CVS, although the evidence is conflicting.

*Ultrasounds.* Ultrasound is used in a variety of ways during a twin gestation. From diagnosis of the multiple gestation to evaluation of the growth patterns of the fetus, the medical community has utilized this tool repeatedly to gain greater insight into the well-being of twin fetuses.

First, ultrasound can be used for a confirmation of multiple gestation, gestational age, chorionicity (optimal timing is 10-14 weeks gestation), fetal sexes (helpful to determine zygosity) and placement of the placenta (Barrett & Bocking, 2000; Tharpe et al., 2013). The medical standard 18-22 week ultrasound can also be used to check for fetal anomalies, which occur more frequently than in singleton pregnancies (Devoe, 2008; Morin & Lim, 2011; Sperling & Tabor, 2001).

Second, nuchal translucency screening done by ultrasound is still valid in multiple gestations, which could reduce the need for amniocentesis in parents with concerns about possible Down's Syndrome (Morin & Lim, 2011; Sperling & Tabor, 2001). This test must be done between 11-13 weeks gestation to be accurate (Fraser et al., 2003, p. 395).

Another common use of ultrasound in twin pregnancies is to determine chorionicity of the fetuses. Ideal gestational timing for assessing chorion status is 10-14 weeks of gestation. Although knowledge of the type of chorion is predictive of possible complications of and necessary counseling for the pregnancy, no studies have shown any difference in pregnancy outcome with foreknowledge of chorionicity (Barrett & Bocking, 2000).

In addition, the medical community utilizes routine, serial ultrasounds at 24, 28, and 32 weeks and thereafter every 2-4 weeks to assess for fetal growth patterns, mainly checking for difference in abdominal circumference between the two fetuses (see Discordant Growth section) (Devaseelan & Ong, 2010; Sperling & Tabor, 2001). Even though this recommendation is done by consensus using studies about differences in fetal growth patterns, no evidence has shown that this practice directly affects pregnancy outcome (Barrett & Bocking, 2000).

Other uses of ultrasound are discussed below in the sections on specific concerns during twin gestation.

***Concerns about ultrasounds.*** Important to note is the latest research on possible concerns about the use of ultrasound in pregnancy. Reporting on the work of Dr. Manuel Casanova, Margulis

> Minicolumns are responsible for higher cognitive functions like facial recognition, joint attention (if I turn my face and look somewhere, a child will turn and look too. Not because I told the child to look, but because the normal human brain is wired to do so), and much more. Joint attention is one of the many qualities that appear to be abnormal in the brains of autistic children (Margulis, 2013, p. 48).

(2013) explains the most recent findings on fetal brain development and autism. In investigating the brains of autistic children, Casanova discovered that fetal brain cells migrate into what scientists are now calling "minicolumns." (See box on previous page.)

As fetal brain cells migrate into these columns, other, complimentary brain cells contain the columns and prevent the columns from spilling into other parts of the brain (Williams & Casanova, 2011). Casanova found that children with autism have a 10-12 percent higher number of minicolumns than neurotypical children. Although no damage to individual neurons has ever been found in babies exposed to prenatal ultrasound, Casanova's hypothesis is that "prolonged or inappropriate ultrasound exposure may actually trigger these cells to divide, migrate and form too many minicolumns. They divide when they're not supposed to and there are no inhibitory cells to contain them" (Margulis, 2013, p. 49; see also Williams & Casanova, 2010).

Definitive cause and effect have not been established, nor has a specific gestational timing of ultrasounds and its impact on fetal neuron migration been determined. However, it would seem prudent to use caution and advise twin gestation clients of the latest research on the possible benefits and risks of using ultrasound in pregnancy.

**Term twin gestation and timing of delivery.** Timing of birth in twin pregnancies is a subject of ongoing research. In general, 37-38 weeks gestation is considered term for twin pregnancy, with the likelihood of stillbirth increasing from that point forward (Cruikshank, 2007; Devaseelan & Ong, 2010). From 39 weeks onward, research has shown the risk of stillbirth exceeds the risk of neonatal death and prolonged twin gestation is considered to occur at 40 weeks (Leveno & Alexander, 2013).

Nutritional considerations affect optimal gestational age in twins, too. In her Multiples Clinic, Dr. Barbara Luke (2011) found that twins whose growth rate is in the lowest ten percent are five times more likely to be born before 33 weeks. Similarly, researchers in Japan

studying outcomes of almost 200,000 twins born in the 1990s found that the combination of optimal gestational age and ideal birth weight was the biggest predictor of mortality and neonatal outcomes with twins (Kato & Matsuda, 2006).

Optimal timing of twin deliveries also needs to account for chorion and amnion status. Due to the severe complications with monoamniotic pregnancies and births (cord entanglements and high mortality), delivery is usually considered around 34 weeks, thus outside the purview of midwives (Barrett & Bocking, 2000; Devaseelan & Ong, 2010). "Consensus views arising from a twins study group commissioned by the Royal College of Obstetricians and Gynaecologists recommend delivery by 37–38 weeks of gestation for dichorionic twins and by 36–37 weeks in uncomplicated monochorionic [, diamniotic] pregnancies" (Devaseelan & Ong, 2010, p. 183).

- Babies who are well nourished in utero have significantly higher birthweights and are healthier at birth than less well-nourished babies born at the same gestational age.
- Good intrauterine nutrition may reduce the likelihood of premature birth. Evidence suggests some survival mechanism detects when babies are not growing well in the womb and may trigger labor. (For instance, twins whose rate of growth during pregnancy is among the lowest 10 percent are five times more likely to be born before 33 weeks...)
- Even if they are born prematurely, babies who have been properly nourished in the womb have fewer illnesses and recover from them more quickly than do infants whose mothers had inadequate diets.
- Because the prenatal period involves the most rapid growth of the entire life cycle, optimal nutrition now provides your babies with the best blueprint for a healthy childhood... (Luke & Eberlein, 2011, pp. 53-54).

**Nutrition in twin gestation.** If nutrition as a hallmark of midwifery care is front and center for most midwives in their care of singleton pregnancies, diet is that much more important in the care of mothers carrying twins. Luke and Eberlein (2011), in their book, *When You're Expecting Twins, Triplets or Quads*, make the points in the box on the previous page.

Hence, a midwife's knowledge of and instruction about nutrition and weight gain can make an enormous difference in the outcomes of pregnancy and delivery for a mother with twins.

Before diving into the differing advice that exists on multiple pregnancies and nutrition, we need to be very clear that definitive evidence for one type of approach to eating for two is nonexistent. In fact, a recent review of all the existing studies on the topic came to one conclusion:

...in aiming "to identify quality controlled studies that compared special diets with normal diets, [they] found none. That is, there is no evidence from randomised trials to advise whether specific dietary advice for women with multiple pregnancies does more good than harm" (Ballard, Bricker, Reed, Wood, & Neilson, 2011, p. 2).

Dietary advice for twin pregnancies ranges from simple requirements (increased calories and iron supplementation with a prenatal multivitamin supplement) to full checklists (with how many servings to eat per day of various food groups, supplementation protocols, and nutrient guidelines) (Brewer, 2013; Luke & Eberlein, 2011; Star, Shannon, Lommel, & Gutierrez, 1999; Weston A. Price Foundation (WAPF), 2004). Most of the diets discussed in these pages have some controversy surrounding them, which will be addressed. The discussion revolves around the controversies, but the actual diet plans shown are the original plans with no changes. Like all things over the course of midwifery care, nutritional advice must weigh the risks and benefits, "providing the mother with individualized education, counseling, and prenatal care" and then deciding together which course is best (Midwifery Task Force, 2008).

***General guidelines.*** In *Ambulatory Obstetrics*, general instruction for nutritional support during a twin gestation include an additional 300 calories above single pregnancy recommendations, prenatal multivitamin and mineral supplement (including 1mg folic acid), and iron supplementation of 60-100mg/day depending on client's hemoglobin status (Star et al., 1999). *Varney's Midwifery's* guidelines differ slightly, only recommending an additional 500 calories and 25 extra grams of protein over the calculated nutrition recommendations for a singleton pregnancy (Varney et al., 2004). The authors also recommend recalculating nutrient requirements at 20 weeks, 28 weeks and 36 weeks of pregnancy (Varney et al., 2004, p. 608).

***Brewer pregnancy diet.*** Touted as a diet to prevent preeclampsia, the *Brewer Diet for Healthy Pregnancy* (2013) gives a checklist of food to eat with other guidelines on salt and water (see http://www.therealblueribbonbaby.org/brewer-diet-checklists/). Anecdotally, there are stories of 9lb+ babies with shoulder dystocia and women who still develop preeclampsia/eclampsia/HELLP while on the diet ("Brewer Diet," 2005; Herrera, 2012). Criticism of the diet comes from views that protein intake is excessive for pregnancy (thereby growing unreasonably large babies) and that, if the diet fails to prevent preeclampsia, the woman feels somehow at fault for not following the diet correctly instead of acknowledging that the diet may not do what it was represented to do.

However, after the diet was developed in 2003, newer research suggests that an inflammatory process is at work in preeclampsia (Major, Campbell, Silver, Branch, & Weyrich, 2014; Odibo, Patel, Spitalnik, Odibo, & Huettner, 2014). It may be that the focus on whole, nutritious foods and seafood with its omega-3 content helps to mitigate the inflammatory processes in developing preeclampsia and, therefore, is of assistance to some women. As for the excess protein issue and big babies, in light of other diet plans for twin gestations, the

Brewer Diet recommendations of 100g-125g of protein in the case of twin pregnancy are in line with other guidelines.

**WAPF *diet for pregnant and nursing mothers.*** This diet plan (see Appendix B) was developed by the Weston A. Price Foundation (WAPF) based on the research of Weston A. Price, a dentist who studied tribal cultures and analyzed their diet and their health, including lack of cavities, full, wide palates and general well-being. He noticed these tribal cultures had different nutritional protocols for expecting mothers than for the general population. Examining the nutrient quality of the food they consumed, he developed dietary recommendations for modern man. His foundation's diet plan for pregnant women comes from this research.

The very first line of the diet plan starts with controversy. Anyone familiar with modern obstetric care is well aware of the standard recommendation to not to exceed a 10,000IU limit of actual Vitamin A (retinol) intake (Rothman et al., 1995). However, several issues remain with this recommendation. First, the study itself did not differentiate between retinol from supplements (typically synthetic) versus retinol contained in actual food, simply grouping both together in their analysis of the birth defects found. Additionally, several letters to the journal's editors take the authors to task (Brent, Hendrickx, Holmes, & Miller, 1996; Challem, 1996; Watkins, Moore, & Mulinare, 1996). They point out that the mean retinol intake of mothers of children born with birth defects was 21,675IU (not the recommended 10,000IU), the number of birth defects ascertained is the same as the population as a whole (which would indicate not all, if any, defects were a result of retinol toxicity), and that the authors' definition of the particular type of defects analyzed created too broad a classification to be attributed to retinol overdose alone. As the WAPF diet gets its retinol from strictly food sources, the problems with the study make it difficult to apply the 10,000IU retinol recommendation accurately in this case. However, the controversy over this issue with cod liver oil is worth discussing with clients to ensure they understand the risks and evidence before following the WAPF diet. Other disputes with the diet include its preference for raw milk, liver, and seafood, in which case, if proper sourcing of the food can be guaranteed, benefits may outweigh risks for clients.

*Dr. Luke's multiples clinic diet plan.* The diet plan covered in Dr. Barbara Luke's book, *When You're Expecting Twins, Triplets and Quads* (2011), is more faceted than the preceding diets. Covering calorie, macronutrient, food group and supplement recommend-ations, the results seen in her clinic establish the quality of her program. Compared to average twins born in the United States, twins born to clients at her clinic are 20% heavier, and more pregnancies are carried to term. The newborns were also less likely to be developmentally delayed in relation to normal twins of the same gestational age (Luke et al., 2003). Although some midwives are of the opinion that supplements of any form should not be required as long as food intake, in both quantity and quality, is high enough, a good case is made from Dr. Luke's clinic outcomes to suggest otherwise in the case of twin pregnancies (Luke, 2005a, 2005b).

Eating every 90 minutes is recommended to deal with the shrinking area available to fill a stomach while trying to meet the daily guidelines. Whole foods are preferred, but nutrient intake takes priority, including advice on utilizing nutritional protein drink and other dietary supplements to add calories and fulfill the diet's nutrient requirements if food intake is inadequate.

Macronutrient requirements for the clinic's diet include calories at 3500 kcal, with protein 20% (176g), carbohydrates 40% (350g) and fat 40% (155g) (Luke & Eberlein, 2011, p. 73). The breakdown of the macronutrients into food groups can be found in Table 1. Daily supplements round out the recommendations for this diet (see Table 2).

More education on multiple pregnancy, as well as guidelines for water, specific menu directions, exercise and other facets of thriving with a twin pregnancy are presented in the book. If clients opt to use

Table 1

*Recommended Daily Servings for Twin Gestation*

| Food Group | Serving Size | Servings |
|---|---|---|
| Dairy | 8 oz. milk<br>8 oz. calcium-fortified cottage cheese<br>8 oz. ice cream<br>1 oz sliced cheese | 8 |
| Vegetables | 1/2 cup cooked or 1 cup fresh | 4 |
| Fruits | 1/2 cup or 1 fresh | 7 |
| Grains, Breads | 1 oz, 1 cup cooked, or 1 slice | 10 |
| Fats, oils, and Nuts | 1 tsp oil<br>1 tsp butter<br>1 oz nuts | 6 |
| Eggs | 1 fresh | 2 |
| Meat, fish, poultry | 3 oz | 3 |

*Note.* Adapted from Luke, B., & Eberlein, T. (2011). *When you're expecting twins, triplets, or quads: Proven guidelines for a healthy multiple pregnancy* (3rd ed.). New York: Harper. p.110. Copyright © 2004 by Dr. Barbara Luke and Tamara Eberlein. Reprinted with permission.

this diet/lifestyle plan during their pregnancy, it is highly recommended they have a copy of the book to reference frequently.

Whatever the diet plan or formulation chosen by the midwife and clients, it seems imperative to understand that one of the most crucial factors in a successful outcome for both mother and babies (and a factor over which some parents can exercise control) is the detail and attention paid to the nutritional intake during pregnancy. Midwives would be wise to follow up about diet at every appointment of twin

Table 2

*Suggested Daily Supplement Regimen*

| Dosage per Tablet | Trimester | | |
|---|---|---|---|
| | First | Second | Third |
| Non-pregnant RDA Multivitamin | 1 tablet | 2 tablets | 2 tablets |
| Calcium/ magnesium/ zinc - 333mg/ 133mg/5mg | 9 tablets | 9 tablets | 9 tablets |
| 1,000mg Vitamin C | 1 tablet | 1 tablet | 1 tablet |
| 400IU Vitamin E | 1 tablet | 1 tablet | 1 tablet |

*Note:* Adapted from Luke, B., & Eberlein, T. (2011). *When you're expecting twins, triplets, or quads: Proven guidelines for a healthy multiple pregnancy (3rd ed.).* New York: Harper. p.76. Copyright © 2004 by Dr. Barbara Luke and Tamara Eberlein. Reprinted with permission.

mothers to ensure clients understand the importance of, and adherence to, the selected nutritional plan for their pregnancy.

**Weight gain.** Weight gain recommendations for twin pregnancies remain highly controversial. In 2009, the United States Institutes of Medicine (IOM) released revised guidance for weight gain in all pregnancies, including specific recommendations for multiple fetuses (National Research Council, 2009). However, this direction was based only on a few studies by Barbara Luke and her colleagues using a single cohort of women (as cited in Siega-Riz, Deierlein, & Stuebe, 2010). Despite this limitation, Dr. Luke's multiples clinic has seen better outcomes, on average, than multiples outside of her clinic. Table 3 compares both the IOM and Dr. Luke's weight gain recommendations for twin pregnancies. Dr. Luke's weight gain guidelines also put

Table 3

*Weight Gain Recommendations in Twin Gestation Based on Beginning Body Mass*

| Body Mass Index (BMI) | IOM | Dr. Luke |
| --- | --- | --- |
| Underweight (BMI < 20) | n/a | 50-66 lbs |
| Normal (BMI 20-24.9) | 37-54 lbs | 40-56 lbs |
| Overweight (BMI 25-29.9) | 31-50 lbs | 38-47 lbs |
| Obese (BMI > 29.9) | 25-42 lbs | 31-36 lbs |

*Note.* BMI may be calculated using a person's height and weight at http:// www.nhlbi.nih.gov/health/educational/lose_wt/BMI/bmicalc.htm IOM = United States Institutes of Medicine Adapted from National Research Council. (2009). *Weight gain during pregnancy: Reexamining the guidelines.* Washington, DC: The National Academies Press and Luke, B., & Eberlein, T. (2011). *When you're expecting twins, triplets, or quads: Proven guidelines for a healthy multiple pregnancy (3rd ed.).* New York: Harper.

forward the idea that the majority of weight be put on by the 28th week of gestation. After this point, she notes that the increasing size of the babies limits the amount of nutrition a woman can physically consume (Luke & Eberlein, 2011). Her weight gain targets for normal weight women pregnant with twins are 25 lbs by 20 WGA (weeks gestational age), and 38 lbs by 28 WGA, with total weight gain being 40-56 lbs and an average gestational length for twins of 36 weeks (Luke & Eberlein, 2011, p. 60).

It is also important to remember that, if weight gain is beneficial to outcomes, more is not necessarily better. Gavard and Artal (2014) found that increasing weight gain over 42 lbs for obese women in term twin pregnancies led to higher risk of preeclampsia and cesarean delivery. In addition, excessive maternal weight gain has been linked to postpartum diabetes and cardiac and other health issues associated with increased BMI (due to increased difficulty in losing the gained gestational weight postnatally).

**Prenatal education.** If a singleton pregnancy and birth changes a women's life forever, surely being pregnant with twins alters the family's life even more so. Physically, the discomforts are more drastic, planning more intense, finances more impacted and learning curve more steep. Greater emphasis on education during pregnancy can help parents understand and prepare for the extraordinary changes that are about to happen.

A midwife's prenatal education checklist should be adapted to include items relevant to mothers pregnant with twins (see Appendix C for possible discussion checklist additions and changes appropriate for twin gestations). She should consider discussing childbirth education options sooner (twin-specific classes can be found in most metropolitan areas) and have readily available resources specific to twins, such as support groups like the National Organization of Mothers of Twins Clubs, for the help with the logistics of double parenting, and La Leche League leaders/IBCLCs with experience in supporting the breastfeeding of twins. Diet should be discussed at every visit, not just a couple of times during pregnancy. Community resources, for example, the government Women, Infants and Children (WIC) program and clinical social workers, can help as mothers adapt to life with two babies. Although bed rest has not been shown to prevent preterm labor, increasing rest time and decreasing work time as the pregnancy progresses allows limited calories to go toward baby growth and helps mothers curb exhaustion and edema from standing (Brubaker & Gyamfi, 2012). Also important to consider is encouraging parents to examine the many possible outcomes of a twin pregnancy, both those good and those involving serious morbidity and mortality.

## Prenatal Complications in Twin Gestation

Complications in twin pregnancies fall into two categories: (1) issues that also occur in singleton pregnancies; and (2) issues that are specific to twin gestation. These complications can include morning sickness and hyperemesis gravidarum, anemia, hypertensive disorders, gestational diabetes mellitus, miscarriage (of one or both fetuses), fetal anomalies, discordant growth and intrauterine growth retardation, and specific issues for monochorionic pregnancies, like twin-to-twin transfusion syndrome and twin reverse arterial perfusion. Remember that, while many difficulties can be prevented with excellent adherence to good nutrition and prenatal care, complications do develop regardless of quality midwifery care or a client's diligence to follow recommendations. Such difficulties must be addressed as circumstances warrant, without fault or blame.

**Maternal responses to pregnancy.** Many standard issues in pregnancy occur at a higher rate in twin gestations. In twin pregnancies, maternal physiological adaptations are more pronounced. From more blood supply, morning sickness and hormones to increased "minor complications of pregnancy such as backache, edema, varicose veins, reflux, hemorrhoids, etc...," twin mothers experience more acute changes than in singletons pregnancies (Edmonds, 2007, p. 169).

*Morning sickness and hyperemesis gravidarum.* Both morning sickness and hyperemesis gravidarum (HG) occur with more severity and more frequency in twin pregnancies (Edmonds, 2007). HG is characterized by persistent nausea and vomiting that usually lasts beyond the first trimester, and is associated with ketosis and weight loss greater than 5% from pre-pregnancy weight (Tharpe et al., 2013). It can lead to dehydration, electrolyte imbalance, acidosis, emotional upheaval, hypokalemia, and alkalosis. Lack of treatment can cause hepatic and renal involvement that can progress to coma and death (Fraser et al., 2003).

Typical morning sickness can be managed conservatively using ginger (250mg QID); peppermint tea; foods rich in B vitamins; acupressure via wristbands; taking bland, high protein foods and complex carbohydrates every two hours to avoid blood sugar drops; increasing sleep, rest and fresh air; and avoiding triggers such as strong odors, heat and stuffy rooms (Tharpe et al., 2013, p. 72). Sometimes, vitamin B6 (with or without Unisom SleepTabs) is used to control symptoms (see Tharpe et al., 2013 for dosages).

For HG, however, IV fluids and/or prescription medications may be needed to alleviate and control symptoms. For dehydration issues, Tharpe et al. (2013) recommends using normal saline for IV hydration, whereas 5% dextrose is recommended in Varney's Midwifery to resolve accompanying ketosis (Varney et al., 2004). If symptoms cannot be alleviated, a physician should be consulted for further evaluation and management.

*Anemia.* Anemia is defined as hemoglobin (Hgb) concentration <11.0g/dL in the first and third trimesters and Hgb < 10.5g/dL in the second trimester (Leveno & Alexander, 2013; Tharpe et al., 2013). In twin pregnancies, red blood cells increase by 300mL more than in singleton pregnancies (Edmonds, 2007). Due to this increase, 40% of twin mothers will experience complete depletion of their iron stores, and some sources recommend all twin mothers be put on iron supplementation. Further, one study showed a 20-30% increased risk of stillbirth in twin pregnancies among anemic mothers (Shumpert, Salihu, & Kirby, 2004).

Because anemia is more prevalent in multiple pregnancies, UK recommendations include hemoglobin testing at 20-24 weeks to identify a need for early supplementation, as well as the standard initial complete blood count (CBC) and Hgb testing at 28 weeks (National Institute of Health and Care Excellence (NICE), 2011).

Although the most common cause of anemia is iron depletion, B12 deficiency and Folic Acid deficiency are also frequently suspect. A CBC lab and thorough diet history can be utilized to narrow the reason(s) for the anemia. Iron-rich foods include green leafy vegetables, collard greens, red meat, egg yolks, raisins, prunes, liver, and blackstrap molasses. Standard supplementation for anemia is 60-120mg of elemental iron daily (Tharpe et al., 2013). Floradix and Hemaplex, both over-the-counter (OTC) supplements, anecdotally produce less gastrointestinal upset than standard iron salts. Once anemia is corrected, recommendations suggest continuing supplementation for at least 3 months to replenish maternal irons stores and suggest continuous dosing through 3 months postpartum (Leveno & Alexander, 2013; Tharpe et al., 2013).

*Hypertensive disorders of pregnancy.* Gestational hypertension and preeclampsia are two to three times more prevalent in twin versus singleton gestations and more likely to be more severe earlier in pregnancy and delivered preterm due to complications of the disease (Edmonds, 2007; Henry, McElrath, & Smith, 2013; Young & Wylie, 2012). HELLP syndrome includes the same findings (Norwitz, Edusa, & Park, 2005). No evidence suggests differing rates of occurrence between monochorionic and dichorionic pregnancies (Edmonds, 2007).

Theories vary on the cause of preeclampsia. On the one hand, the medical consensus is that the "pathological hallmark of preeclampsia is shallow endovascular invasion of the placenta" (Norwitz et al., 2005, p. 343). In other words, the placenta has a shallow implantation.

Alternatively, preeclampsia can develop in women with chronic inflammation, causing speculation on causal theories of low omega-3 fetal brain fat supplies, which is supported by the disappearance of preeclampsia symptoms after the fetal demise of one twin (Borzychowski, Sargent, & Redman, 2006; Norwitz et al., 2005; Odent, 2001). Odent (2001) points out that,

> in preeclampsia, the level of DHA is not significantly decreased, whereas the level of the parent molecule EPA is about 10 times lower than in normal pregnancy…[Therefore,] theoretically, the most direct way to prevent preeclampsia would be to consume sea fish that is rich in n-3 polyunsaturates and also in minerals that are essential nutrients for the brain (eg, iodine, selenium, and zinc) (pp. 3, 5).

This theory supports the United Kingdom recommendation that women pregnant with twins take 75mg of aspirin daily, from 12 weeks gestation until delivery, if they have one or more of the following risk factors for developing a hypertensive disorder: (1) first pregnancy, (2) age 40 or over, (3) pregnancy interval of more than 10 years, (4) BMI of 35 kg/m2 or more at the first visit or (5) family history of preeclampsia (National Institute of Health and Care Excellence (NICE), 2011). In addressing the aspirin recommendation, Odent (2001) points out that the anti-platelet effect of aspirin intervenes late in the chain of events (from his n-3 oil theory), halting the cascade leading to preeclampsia and other hypertensive disorders.

Regardless, Varney et al.'s (2004) admonition that "close observation of blood pressure measurement, weight gain, proteinuria, and edema in addition to development of headaches and scotomata" be rigorously honored is good advice. (p. 693)

***Gestational diabetes.*** Gestational Diabetes Mellitus (GDM) is curious different in twin gestation. Incidence is thought to be slightly increased in multiple gestation, with one source reporting an occurrence rate of 5% - 8% of twin pregnancies and another giving a 3.98% rate compared to 2.32% rate for single pregnancies (Norwitz et al., 2005; Rauh-Hain et al., 2009; Santolaya & Faro, 2012; Varney et al., 2004). Other sources find a similar incidence of GDM in twin gestation as in single pregnancies with Young & Wylie (2012) postulating that, although a larger placental mass increases amounts of placental steroid hormones circulating in twin gestation mothers, similar insulin levels required in single and twin GDM pregnancies suggest that GDM is no more severe a complication in multiple gestation than in single pregnancies (Buhling et al., 2003). Simoes et al. (2011) found that incidence of GDM in twin gestation is possibly related to presence of pre-gravid maternal obesity with Rauh-Hain et al. (2009) finding the highest risks for twin GDM exists in African-Americans and young women.

However, outcomes, when compared to their single gestation GDM counterparts, find almost a helpful, possibly "compensatory" status to GDM in twin pregnancies (Cruz, Foeller, Zhao, & Szabo, 2014). Research shows reduced risks for many adverse outcomes such as lower (up to 50% less) neonatal death, less depressed 5-minute APGAR scores, and less small for gestational age (SGA) with no difference in large for gestational age (LGA) or macrosomia when compared to non-diabetic twin gestations (Cruz et al., 2014; Guillen et al., 2014). Weight discrepancy between twin A and twin B was found to be either the same or actually less (when GDM is managed with insulin) compared with higher rates of weight discrepancies in non-GDM twins at birth (Guillen et al., 2014; Klein, Mailath-Pokorny, Leipold, Krampl-Bettelheim, & Worda, 2010). In addition, Guillen et al. (2014) found that weight discrepancy rates were not influenced by glycemic control in GDM twin mothers.

The body of literature on twin pregnancy does indicate a few risks that are slightly higher in GDM twin pregnancies when compared to non-GDM twin pregnancies. Increased neonatal intensive care (NICU) admission, increased incidence of respiratory distress syndrome (RDS) along with longer hospitalization were found in mother with GDM in a few studies (Rauh-Hain et al., 2009; Simoes et al., 2011). Importantly, in two large-scale comparison studies, even though risk of GDM is similar in single and twin gestation, presence of GDM, only in twin gestation, was highly associated with increased risk for gestational hypertension and preeclampsia (Buhling et al., 2003; Guillen et al., 2014).

*Management of GDM.* Management of GDM in twin gestation is currently recommended to be the same as in singleton gestation. After reviewing the one step, 75 gram diagnostic glucose tolerance test (GTT) in 2013, the National Institutes of Health (NIH) recommended that practitioners in the US stay with the two step, 50 gram glucose challenge test followed by the 100 gram GTT for diagnosis of gestational diabetes (Metzger et al., 2007; Vandorsten et al., 2013). Diagnosing GDM is just as in a singleton pregnancy, with the normative values remaining the same: see Vandorsten et al. (2013) for protocols and values.

Once diagnosed, diet and/or insulin therapy with blood glucose monitoring are the standard method of treatment. Oral hypoglycemics (metformin, glyburide) have been studied in single gestation, but not enough evidence exists to inform their use in twin pregnancy per se.

Alternative measures to include cinnamon (1/4 to 1/2 tsp daily), bilberry, chicory, dandelion, and red raspberry (Romm, 2003; Tharpe et al., 2013).

Gymnema, although a powerful herb in regards to sugar metabolism, is listed as a uterine tonic (like red raspberry) in some places and as a constituent in herbal preparations to activate the uterus in others (Tiwari, Mishra, & Sangwan, 2014). Accordingly, use in pregnancy should take into account possible "uterine activation."

**Miscarriage and single intrauterine fetal demise.** (See also Fetal Anomalies and Preterm Labor.) Miscarriage and intrauterine fetal death complications show an inherent difference in normalcy along trimester and chorionicity dividing lines. Death of a single fetus in occurs in 3.7% - 6.8% of twin pregnancies and can occur at any time, with a 13.8% risk in monoamniotic gestation before week 22 gradually decreasing to 4.5%-8.0% between week 30 and 36 (Blickstein & Perlman, 2013; Morikawa, Yamada, Yamada, Sato, & Minakami, 2012).

Reasons for fetal demise in twin gestation include etiology normal to any pregnancy (genetic and anatomical issues, growth restriction, placental insufficiency, etc.) and those specific to twin gestation, primarily among monoamniotic and monochorionic gestations (TTTS and cord entanglement concerns). As in single pregnancies, the reason behind fetal death often remains unknown. Management of the fetal demise depends on whether a full spontaneous abortion of the affected fetus occurs and implications of the death on the remaining co-twin.

Most early fetal deaths result in "vanishing twin syndrome" and can occur as late as the end of the first trimester. Vaginal bleeding, in such cases, can occur without any products of conception being expelled. In dichorionic (DC) pregnancies, it is probably harmless to the surviving co-twin and the twin may be completely reabsorbed or become a fetus papyraceus (Blickstein & Perlman, 2013; Norwitz et al., 2005). In MC pregnancies, although probably just as harmless to the surviving co-twin, the mechanism of demise may include TTTS issues and/or twin reversed arterial perfusion (TRAP) sequence that cannot be seen, so an ultrasound and possibly third-trimester MRI may be warranted to evaluate the co-twin for possible brain and kidney abnormalities (Blickstein & Perlman, 2013). Continuing midwifery care in these cases, after consultation, may be justified.

Fetal demise and/or miscarriage in the second and third trimester become more problematic for midwifery care in a twin pregnancy. Risk factors vary in these cases. Timing of a fetal demise was found to be inversely related to survival of the co-twin at one year of age. The earlier the demise occurred after 20 weeks, the more likely the co-twin would survive to age one year (Johnson & Zhang, 2002). Opposite gender between the twins also increased survival rates.

If a complete spontaneous abortion occurs after the fetal demise, the remaining fetus will usually be delivered within 3 weeks, although this can vary and be as long as 18 weeks (Adamowicz, Przybylkowska,

Trzeciak-Supel, & Filipp, 2004; D'Antonio, Khalil, Dias, Thilaganathan, & Southwest Thames Obstetric Research, 2013). Emergency cerclage has been found to postpone the delivery interval and give time for further development of the remaining co-twin (Petousis et al., 2012).

In cases of second and third trimester fetal demise, consult from, if not complete transfer of care to, an obstetrician is completely warranted. For DC pregnancies, disseminated intravascular coagulation (DIC) does not seem to be an issue, although evaluation of Rh-mothers, just as in other miscarriages, is justified (Blickstein & Perlman, 2013). But increased risk of infection from a completed spontaneous abortion, possibility of very preterm labor, and need for steroids to hasten lung development place management of these pregnancies outside of the scope of midwifery. Also, for remaining MC co-twins, the increased incidence of co-twin demise and, if surviving to delivery, neurodevelopment issues place these pregnancies at higher risk and affirm the need for increased surveillance by obstetricians and/or maternal-fetal specialists (Hillman, Morris, & Kilby, 2011).

No matter the outcome, in all cases of fetal demise, care should be taken to assist the parents in getting bereavement counseling and any other mental health services required.


**Fetal anomalies.** Compared to singleton pregnancies, twin gestations have a 70% higher rate of congenital abnormalities (when including conjoined and acardiac twins, covered in the Complications specific to Twin Gestation subsection below) (Glinianaia, Rankin, & Wright, 2008). One study showed the rate of malformations at 8.9% in monochorionic twins and 6.1% in dichorionic twins while another study showed the rate of anomalies nearly double in MC twins compared to DC twins (Glinianaia et al., 2008; Lato, Berg, Gembruch, & Geipel, 2009). The Scottish Stillbirth and Neonatal Death Report gave a perinatal death rate of 1.98/1000 among multiples, double the rate for singletons (Twining, McHugo, & Pilling, 2007).

Cardiac defects are some of the most prevalent among MC twins with a reported rate of 18.9/1000 compared to 7.4/1000 among DC twins and 6/1000 among singletons (Twining et al., 2007). Rates in the United Kingdom among monozygotic twins are reported to be as high as 32/1000 (Fraser et al., 2003). Some of these defects include transposition errors and ventricular septal defects (Glinianaia et al., 2008; Twining et al., 2007). The UK recommendation is that all MC twins receive an echocardiogram at 20 weeks (Fraser et al., 2003). Critical congenital heart defect (CCHD) screening is also crucial in the newborn period for these babies.

On the other hand, more discordant anomalies in DC twins are seen in the central nervous system including neural tube defects like spina bifida, although they occur at a higher rate in both DC and MC twins than in singletons (Glinianaia et al., 2008; Lato et al., 2009). Other congenital anomalies that occur at a greater rate in twins than singletons include tracheo-esophageal fistula (a five-fold increase with 95% discordant for the abnormality), anencephaly, renal dysplasia, hydronephrosis, hydrocephalus, "facial clefts, anomalies of eye, ear, face and neck, anomalies of respiratory, digestive system, syndromes and multiple anomalies" (Glinianaia et al., 2008, p. 1308; see also Lato et al., 2009; Twining et al., 2007).

In terms of chromosomal issues, the rates of anomalies are similar to singleton pregnancies (Glinianaia et al., 2008). Dichorionic babies have twice the maternal age-related risk than monochorionic twins due to the fertilization of two eggs instead of one in such pregnancies, although there is some evidence that Down's Syndrome occurs less frequently in twins than singletons (Edmonds, 2007).

Management of anomalies varies from selective termination of one fetus to expectant management of the pregnancy. In cases of MC anencephaly, the complications of polyhydramnios leading to preterm labor combined with high intra-uterine death rates for the affected twin usually result in a decision of selective termination (Twining et al., 2007). Otherwise, the death of the anencephalic twin will cause the death of the normal co-twin.

In any selective termination, there is always the risk of feticide for the second twin with a loss rate of 7% in the literature (Edmonds, 2007). One study looked at 30 twin pairs discordant for abnormalities (Linskens, Elburg, Oepkes, Vugt, & Haak, 2011). While three pregnancies elected to have selective termination, and two pregnancies had complete terminations, the remaining 25 pregnancies utilized expectant management. Three had spontaneous fetal demise of the affected fetus. The five twins with lethal anomalies opted for non-intervention comfort care at birth and the non-affected twins all had good outcomes. In such cases, coordination of care during pregnancy between pediatricians, obstetrician,s and genetic counselors is needed, as well as utilizing psychological care for the parents.

Diagnosis of such abnormalities is one of the main reasons given for structural and cardiac ultrasounds of twin gestations in the prenatal period. The increased incidence rate combined with the ability to arrange specialized services, if needed, inform parents' choices and decisions. While some parents may decide to decline a prenatal ultrasound, a thorough discussion with parents about the impact and importance (pro and con) of any information gained from an ultrasound screening needs to be part of "providing the mother with individualized education, counseling, and prenatal care" highlighted in the Midwives Model of Care (Midwifery Task Force, 2008).

**Preterm labor.** Prematurity is currently responsible for 70% of neonatal mortality and 25-50% of long-term neurologic impairments in children (American College of Obstetricians and Gynecologists (ACOG) Committee on Practice Bulletins-Obstetrics, 2012). In the case of twin pregnancies, preterm delivery is about six times more likely than in singleton pregnancies, with 45.6% of all twin pregnancies delivering moderately preterm (Lee, Cleary-Goldman, & D'Alton, 2006). Sometimes complications necessitate the delivery of twins in the preterm period, such as intrauterine growth restriction (IUGR) and preeclampsia.

Acute polyhydramnios can be a cause of preterm labor. The

condition exacerbates the distention to the uterus caused by the double fetal load, making the uterus even more susceptible to irritability. Usually caused from other complications such as TTTS and fetal anomalies, it is also more prevalent in MC twins well (Fraser et al., 2003).

Boulet et al. (2008) found that women conceiving twins through artificial reproductive technology (ART) were less likely to be born premature, have a low birthweight or experience infant death in primiparous women (no difference was noted among multiparous women) although another study suggest that ART leads to higher rates of preterm delivery (Luke et al., 2004). In addition, women with lower socioeconomic status were found to have higher rates of preterm twin delivery among other complications (Zhang, Meikle, Grainger, & Trumble, 2002).

For prediction of risk of preterm labor in multiple pregnancies, there are several well-studied options. Risk of preterm labor in twin gestation is increased by previous preterm labor in a singleton pregnancy, teen maternal age, urinary tract infections and shortened cervical length (Brubaker & Gyamfi, 2012; Salihu et al., 2005; Schaaf, Hof, Mol, Abu-Hanna, & Ravelli, 2012).

Premature cervical shortening and cervical funneling detected by transvaginal ultrasound examination have good predictive capabilities for the development of preterm labor and delivery in women with multiple gestations. Studies suggest that a cervical length measurement of greater than or equal to 35 mm at 24 to 26 weeks identifies women with twins who are at low risk for delivery before 34 weeks' gestation. On the other hand, a cervical length of 25 mm or less with or without funneling at 24 weeks' gestation predicts a high risk for preterm labor and delivery. In addition, one study also found that a positive fetal fibronectin test at 28 weeks is a significant predictor of spontaneous preterm labor before 32 weeks' gestation" (Y. Lee et al., 2006, p. 107). Additionally, Tan, Wen, Walker & Demissie (2004) found that a significant risk factor for preterm birth (and other morbidities) among twin deliveries was partial or complete lack of the paternal partner's birth certificate information, indicating an important social factor of which providers need to be cognizant.

Treatments investigated for the prevention of preterm labor, which have not proven beneficial, include prophylactic cervical cerclage, routine bed rest, prophylactic tocolytics, and home uterine monitoring (Y. Lee et al., 2006). However, one recommendation for women with a history of preterm delivery, IUGR, or pregnancy-induced hypertension in a previous pregnancy is daily supplementation with 2.7g of Omega 3 fish oil. One study found a 44% and 39% reduction in spontaneous preterm delivery among low- and middle-level fish consumers, respectively (Olsen et al., 2007). In contrast, though, high-level fish consumers received no benefit from additional Omega-3 intake. Additionally, the study showed supplementation does not confer any benefit with the sole risk factor being a twin gestation. Another treatment being investigated is the use of transvaginal progesterone cream for the prevention of preterm labor in twin gestation. While promising in singleton pregnancies, results have been less definitive in progesterone use with twins. The most promising indication suggests that vaginal progesterone may be beneficial in twin gestations with a short cervix identified by ultrasound between 20 and 25 weeks (Brubaker & Gyamfi, 2012).

**Complications specific to twin gestation.** Particular complications occur due to the nature of the physiology, implantation and/or interaction between the fetuses in twin gestation. These difficulties are not encountered in singleton gestation and should be understood by any midwife contemplating the inclusion of twins in her personal scope of practice.

*Discordant growth and IUGR.* In twins, 16% of those born will have growth discrepancy of 20% or more (Miller, Chauhan, & Abuhamad, 2012). When diagnosing discordant growth, the larger twin is used as the reference with ACOG establishing 15%-25% difference in fetal weight as the definition and the Society of Obstetricians and

Gynaecologists of Canada (SOGC) determining either 20% difference in fetal weight OR 20 mm difference in abdominal circumference as designating growth discordance (Miller et al., 2012).

Discordant growth happens for a variety of reasons with twins, most of which can be categorized by zygosity. Monozygotic twins are usually discordant for growth due to TTTS or the presence of structural anomalies, since genetic material is almost identical between the twins. In dizygotic twins, discordant growth can be due to several reasons. First, basic differences in genetic potential, especially with opposite genders, can lead to a possibly trivial growth discrepancy. Second, implantation differences between the twins can cause the twin with better access to nutrition to grow faster or lead to growth restriction in the other twin. Regardless of the reason, Miller et al. (2012) found that twins with a 25% difference in fetal weight had a higher rates of problems and a fetal weight discordance >30% led to a five-fold increase in fetal death. However, studies show that higher gestational age and increased fetal weight minimize any neonatal complications. For every 1 week increase in gestational age, Frezza et al. (2011) found a significant decrease in all adverse neonatal outcomes related to discordant growth and every 250g increase in fetal weight was found to decrease mortality by 84%. As such, "discordance alone should not be considered as a predictor for adverse neonatal outcome" nor an indication for preterm delivery (Frezza et al., 2011, p. 463; see also Miller et al., 2012).

*Mono (both chorionic and amnionic) twin issues.* Certain conditions occur due to the nature of monozygotic implantation and development. Because of these conditions, once diagnosed, almost all require care outside the scope of a midwife. Indeed, prompt medical intervention can mean the difference between a fulfilling life or a poor quality existence and/or death for one or both twins. Midwives should seriously consider the responsibility involved with monozygotic twins and firmly decide whether these cases warrant inclusion within a midwife's scope of practice, especially for birth in home or birth centers.

*Twin-to-twin transfusion syndrome.* Almost all monochorionic twins have some vascular anomalies in the placenta which are of little consequence. In Twin-to-Twin Transfusion Syndrome (TTTS), however, the anomalies are more significant and allow for transfusion of blood between one twin (the donor) and its sibling (the receiver). Estimates are that TTTS occurs in 25% of MC pregnancies (Leveno & Alexander, 2013). Due to lack of fluid, the donor twin develops oligohydramnios in its separate sac and can develop growth restriction and pulmonary hypoplasia while the recipient is stricken with severe polyhydramnios due to increased urine production from the transfusion of blood. This receiver twin can then progress to cardiac problems and heart failure due to the increased blood volume as well as premature rupture of membranes due to the excess amniotic fluid and possible fetal death. (Gratacos, Ortiz, & Martinez, 2012; Leveno & Alexander, 2013).

The recommendation in the United Kingdom is to scan MC twins every two weeks to check for signs of TTTS with the ideal treatment of laser ablation being performed before 26 weeks gestation (Devaseelan & Ong, 2010; Fraser et al., 2003). The ideal time to diagnose TTTS is between 16 and 24 weeks gestational age, and, after this point, diagnosis is uncommon (Royal College of Obstetricians and Gynaecologists (RCOG), 2008). Once diagnosed, twins with TTTS should be referred to medical care from a maternal-fetal medicine specialist.

*Twin reduced arterial perfusion.* Twin reduced arterial perfusion (TRAP) happens in 1 in every 35,000 births. Occurring in monochorionic pregnancies, a normal twin donates deoxygenated arterial blood via an abnormal placental shunt to a recipient twin. Due to the abnormal structure, this "used" blood typically only perfuses the lower body. Hence, stunted growth and development of the upper half of the recipient's body is the result. Another name for the condition is acardiac twinning due to the lack of development of a heart in the recipient twin (Leveno & Alexander, 2013). Overall, the survival rate of the pump twin with no intervention is 60%, depending on accompanying problems such as polyhydramnios, preterm birth or growth discordance (Devaseelan & Ong, 2010). If radiofrequency ablation of umbilical vessels in the acardiac twin occurs, the survival rate increases to 90% for the pump twin (H. Lee et al., 2007).

*Monoamniotic twin conditions.* Diagnosed via ultrasound when no dividing membrane is visible between the fetuses, monoamniotic pregnancies occur in approximately 1 percent of all monozygotic twins (Leveno & Alexander, 2013). Although cord entanglement (occurring in half of all cases) is considered a major cause of fetal death in these pregnancies, a recent examination by Rossi & Prefumo (2013) concluded that cord entanglements do not contribute to prenatal mortality or morbidity in monoamniotic pregnancies (Leveno & Alexander, 2013; Royal College of Obstetricians and Gynaecologists (RCOG), 2008). It is important to note that most fetal demise due to such cord entanglements happen earlier in pregnancy. Another cord issue to consider with monoamniotic twins include intermittent cord compression (Lee, 2012). Lower incidence occurs once gestation reaches 30-32 weeks and babies have less room to move (Leveno & Alexander, 2013). Still, a retrospective study showed a monoamniotic survival rate of twin pairs of 60% (Royal College of Obstetricians and Gynaecologists (RCOG), 2008).

Conjoined twins also occur in monoamniotic pregnancies. Incidence is rare, with one source citing a rate of 1 in 60,000 pregnancies and another source giving a rate of 1 in 90,000-100,000 pregnancies (Leveno & Alexander, 2013; Royal College of Obstetricians and Gynaecologists (RCOG), 2008). Most instances are diagnosed by ultrasound before 20 weeks of pregnancy and should be referred to competent medical care.

# 5 INTRAPARTUM MANAGEMENT OF TWIN GESTATION

The following section presents a discussion of the current, modern evidence for different practices and procedures during the intrapartum period. In evaluating the literature surrounding facilitation of vaginal birth of twin gestations, there is a serious shortage in what would be considered midwifery "art." Good, descriptive sources of such art can be found on blog posts, Midwifery Today articles and other midwifery resources (see Appendix D for a list of references).

In preparing the management of a twin delivery, "multiple factors should be considered when deciding on the appropriate mode of delivery, including gestational age, fetal lie, estimated fetal weights, provider skills and experience, and patient preference" (Lee, 2012, pp.

Of utmost importance throughout labor and delivery is that the [provider] have a carefully thought-out plan regarding what he or she will do in the event of cord prolapse, placental separation before delivery of the second twin, change in position of the second twin during delivery of the first, immediate postpartum hemorrhage, and other complications (Cruikshank, 2007, p. 1168).

197-198). A midwife must take all these elements into account when consulting with the mother and formulating a best plan for the birth.

## Intrapartum Twin Fetal Surveillance

"Safe care for mothers and babies during labor and birth is the goal of all health care professionals and is an expectation of childbearing women and their families. Fetal assessment is a key aspect of perinatal [client] safety" (Simpson, 2010, p. 1). Midwives need to assure that adequate fetal assessment occurs for both fetuses throughout the labor and birth.

**Staffing.** When attending out-of-hospital birth for twin gestation, the head midwife needs to guarantee enough "hands on deck." At least three, if not four, midwives need to be present: one or two midwives for the mother as well as one midwife per baby. In addition, one or two skilled assistants need to be present to aid and support (Frye, 2004).

**Fetal monitoring.** During labor, midwives should, at a minimum, follow the intermittent auscultation (IA) guidelines given by the ACNM (2010) when assessing fetal well-being. Guidelines suggest checking every hour during latent phase and then every 15-30 minutes during active phase and every 5-15 minutes during pushing. Techniques for IA are also given in the clinical bulletin, including verifying baselines and then determining responses to contractions. Another resource with pertinent information on fetal monitoring is the NICHD Definitions and Classifications: Application to Electronic Fetal Monitoring Interpretation (Simpson, 2010).

Evaluation and charting will need to be done for both babies, possibly at the same time to assure that the midwife, thinking she is examining twin B, is not repeating a check on twin A.

## Considerations of Vaginal Delivery with Twins

When planning a delivery with twins, certain normal consideration of labor and birth have facets unique to twins that must be understood before managing such a birth. Some of these considerations include best place of delivery, vaginal birth after cesarean, placenta previa, cord prolapse, inducing labor, dysfunctional labor patterns, premature rupture of membranes, and bleeding and hemorrhage.

**Place of delivery.** In deliberations with parents about the place of delivery for their twin children, significant consideration should be on research that shows, for the best neonatal outcomes (APGAR scores, seizure occurrence and need for ventilation), the vaginal/ cesarean combination of birth is worse than vaginal birth for both twins or cesarean birth (either planned or in early labor) for both twins (Cruikshank, 2007; Wen et al., 2004). It is not clear whether this is an effect of the reason for the emergency cesarean (cord prolapse or fetal distress, for example) or due to the vaginal/cesarean birth combination itself. If it is possible that twin B may need to come via cesarean, midwives should discuss with clients the benefits and risks of a planned cesarean versus an attempted vaginal birth at home or in the hospital.

**Vaginal birth after cesarean (VBAC).** Most mothers who have had a previous cesarean will choose to have a repeat cesarean when contemplating the delivery of their twins. However, for those choosing a trial of labor after cesarean (TOLAC), the likelihood of a successful VBAC is the same as for mothers with singleton gestations (Leveno & Alexander, 2013). TOLAC has also been found not to increase maternal morbidity, including uterine rupture, nor be an independent risk factor for perinatal mortality (Aaronson, Harlev, Sheiner, & Levy, 2010). Several studies gave the successful VBAC rate for twin deliveries at 65% (Cruikshank, 2007). However, no studies are available to ascertain the risk of uterine rupture with a scarred uterus should a breech extraction of twin B be necessary (Cruikshank, 2007).

The same evaluation criteria apply as for singleton TOLAC, except that a prior vaginal birth has not been shown to significantly increase rates of a successful VBAC in cases of twin gestation (Varner et al., 2005). These criteria should be used in determining feasibility for attempting a VBAC, taking into account the lack of breech extraction data for twin TOLACs.

Although a hospital may be the absolute safest option in such situations, finding a hospital willing to allow a TOLAC for a twin birth is problematic at best. Mothers should be counseled accordingly.

**Placenta previa.** Placenta previa can occur both prenatally and during labor in twin gestations. Prenatally, placenta previa occurs more frequently with dichorionic twins than monochorionic or singleton pregnancies. Diagnosed by ultrasound, such placentae previae normally resolve by 32 weeks gestation (Weis, Harper, Roehl, Odibo, & Cahill, 2012).

Rarely, during labor, the first baby's placenta may become detached from the uterine wall and, as the uterus contracts to pull itself around the second twin, the detached placenta is moved down and covers the internal os. If this occurs, transport is necessary to deliver the second twin unless profuse bleeding requires the second twin to be born immediately by internal version and breech extraction. Care must be taken to ensure that the midwife, feeling along the placental edge while gaining access through the os, finds the loose side of the placenta and does not dislodge the side still attached to the uterine wall, thereby further endangering the second twin (Frye, 2004).

**Cord prolapse.** As in singleton pregnancies, cord prolapse can occur anytime the membranes rupture when a fetus has not descended into the pelvis (Lin, 2006). Hence, it is very important to leave the membranes of twin B intact until baby is fully engaged in the pelvis (Frye, 2004) . Breech, including footling, complete or kneeling breech, as well as transverse, presentations can also lead to cord prolapse (Eleje, Ofojebe, Udegbuman, Adichie, 2014; Frye, 2004). In monoamniotic twins, there is also a chance of cord descending after the birth of the first twin, before the second twin is engaged in the pelvis (Sebire, Snijders, Hughes & Nicolaides, 1997). Although good planning and practice can mitigate (but not eliminate) the chance of a cord prolapse, immediate delivery or transport is required once it occurs (Frye, 2004).

**Inducing labor.** Although midwives promote "natural" childbirth, there can be indications where an induction of labor is necessary. These reasons can range from poor placental grading, maternal hypertension and other factors or even parental preference, such as when mandatory transfer is necessary due to licensing requirements like a gestational age limit for a client remaining in care. Each midwife must decide whether they will accommodate so-called "natural" induction requests or transfer their clients to other medical personnel when these indications arise. One study showed that, while not increasing maternal morbidity, induction of labor in twins is an independent risk factor for the need of a cesarean delivery at a rate of 31% if induction was used and 17% when labor was allowed to start on its own (Okby, Shoham-Vardi, Ruslan, & Sheiner, 2013).

**Dysfunctional labor/prolonged labor patterns.** According to Frye (2004), the active phase of a natural twin labor should be very similar to that of a natural singleton labor; however, the prodromal phase may be extended. Research by Leftwich and her associates (2013) reinforces that observation. They analyzed over 800 twin labors and compared their dilation patterns to those of singleton pregnancies. Twin labors took 2-3 hours longer, on average, than singletons to complete dilation (see Figure 2). The most interesting information, though, is that, unlike multiparous singleton births which are usually faster than their nulliparous counterparts, multiparous twin dilation is actually slower overall than nulliparous twin dilation, with the last part of dilation occurring quickly to give both multiparous and nulliparous twin labors a similar length of time to complete dilation. Another

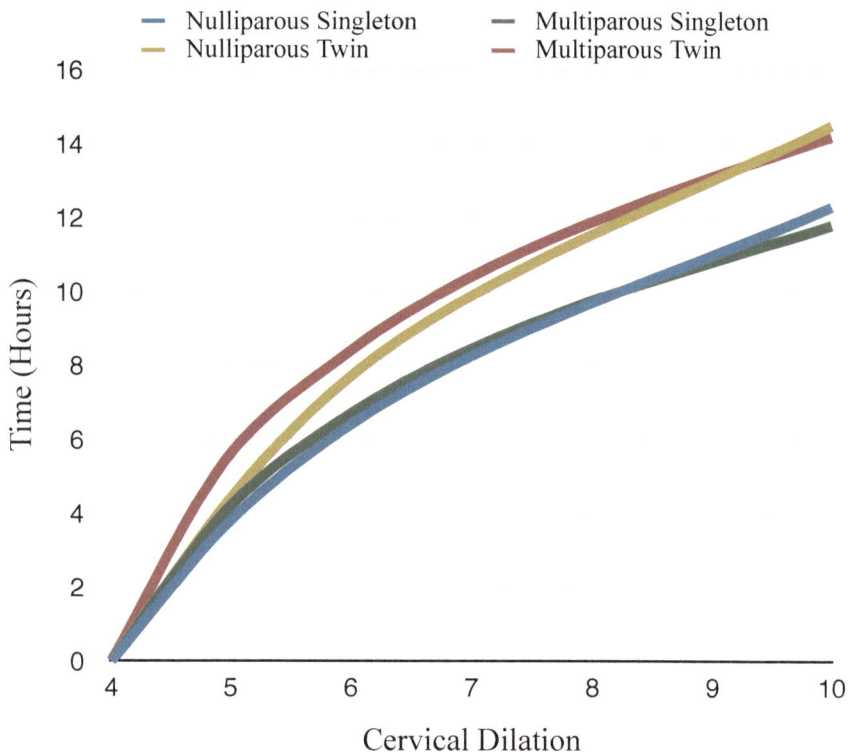

Figure 2. Dilation Curves for Singleton and Twin Gestations. Adapted from Leftwich, H. K., Zaki, M. N., Wilkins, I., & Hibbard, J. U. (2013). Labor patterns in twin gestations. *American Journal of Obstetrics & Gynecology, 209*(3), 254 e251-255.

study showed a similar conclusion (Silver et al., 2000). With new research defining active labor as occurring at 6 cm, this study strengthens that assertion since dilation patterns for both nullipara and multipara are somewhat similar once dilation reaches 6 cm (American College of Obstetricians & Gynecologists et al., 2014).

Sometimes, an extraordinarily distended uterus will not function as efficiently as it should (Frye, 2004). This sign could indicate potential problems further in the progression of labor and postpartum, such as labor completely stalling or postpartum hemorrhage due to uterine atony. If labor does not progress normally, transport is required.

**Premature rupture of membranes (PROM).** Premature rupture of membranes (PROM) comes in two varieties. The first, at term, occurs when membranes rupture before the start of labor. Frye (2004) suggests daily supplementation of Vitamin C with bioflavonoids to strengthen the amniotic sac and prevent rupture before birth. However, a 2010 study on gestational hypertension was abruptly halted early when "vitamin C and E supplementation did not reduce the rate of preeclampsia or [gestational hypertension], but increased the risk of fetal loss or perinatal death and preterm prelabor rupture of membranes" (Xu et al., 2010). That result may be due to the vitamin E included in the study as other current research supported Frye's assertion (Ghomian, Hafizi, & Takhti, 2013; Osaikhuwuomwan, Okpere, Okonkwo, Ande, & Idogun, 2011).

The second, preterm premature rupture of membranes (PPROM), occurs before term. In twin pregnancies, PPROM occurs in about 7%-8% of all twin pregnancies, at an average of 30 - 32 weeks gestation, with studies suggesting a shorter time until labor begins with twins compared with singletons experiencing PPROM, with twins averaging 24 hours until delivery and most delivered by 7 days post PPROM (Sela & Simpson, 2011). If PPROM occurs before term, transfer of care is necessary as medical interventions, such as tocolytics, antenatal steroids and antibiotic therapy, can decrease neonatal morbidity if started early.

In a recent article, different explanations were evaluated as to the cause of PPROM. Looking at infection/inflammation, placental bleeding, uterine over-distention, and genetic variations, the authors hypothesized that all these factors overlap and work synergistically to weaken membranes and cause rupture before term (Lannon, Vanderhoeven, Eschenbach, Gravett, & Adams Waldorf, 2014). Indeed, several studies have implicated group beta strep infections as a cause of PROM (Gibbs, Romero, Hillier, Eschenbach, & Sweet, 1992;

Regan, Chao, & James, 1981). Of these factors, very little can be done with genetic variations or placental bleeding. On the other hand, strengthening vaginal flora and infection prevention can be addressed prenatally and extreme uterine over-distention can be influenced with good diet and nutrition (as well as encouraging healthy tissue maintenance). Attention to both of these issues can help assuage the possibility of developing PPROM.

**Bleeding and hemorrhage.** Almost 50 years ago, hemorrhage was given as a common risk for twin pregnancies, occurring in up to 15% of deliveries (O'Sullivan, 1968). With twins, keeping uterine tone is problematic due to the over-distention of the uterus or uterine atony. Also, the large loss of body mass will lead to symptoms of circulatory compromise, if not actual shock, in many mothers (Frye, 2004). When evaluating risk factors for postpartum hemorrhage, Wetta et al. (2013) did not find twins to be an independent risk factor like Hispanic and non-Hispanic white, preeclampsia or chorioamnionitis, but it was a risk factor nonetheless. This finding was echoed in a 2014 study by Wenckus and other researchers who found increased hemorrhage and need for transfusion among women delivering twins. Another study found that, unlike singleton deliveries, twin deliveries with higher risk of hemorrhage included gestational age $\geq 41$ weeks or the presence of hypertensive disorders (Suzuki, Hiraizumi, & Miyake, 2012).

Research into prevention of postpartum hemorrhage in twin births seems to be limited to the use of pharmaceuticals. Several studies (and personal management technique articles) cover use of oxytocin prophylactically to prevent hemorrhage after twin births, with one study showing that 10 units in 500 mL saline solution given intravenously for the first hour just as effective as larger doses (Cruikshank, 2007; Lee, 2012; Tita et al., 2012; Westhoff, Cotter, & Tolosa, 2013). New research is also showing the efficacy of date consumption on labor outcomes. One study analyzed ingestion of 6 dates per day for the last 4 weeks of labor, demonstrating improved outcomes in length of labor, less need for oxytocin and less postpartum hemorrhage among other findings (Al-Kuran, Al-Mehaisen, Bawadi, Beitawi, & Amarin, 2011). Another investigation showed a 50g dose of dates (3-7 dates, depending on size) after delivery was more effective than synthetic oxytocin at reducing postpartum bleeding (Khadem, Sharaphy, Latifnejad, Hammod, & Ibrahimzadeh, 2007). It is worth noting, however, that neither of these date studies was specifically focused on twin delivery.

Although herbal preparations are used frequently postpartum by midwives to prevent blood loss and hemorrhage with good results, lack of current research into their efficacy makes it difficult to recommend them as a viable therapy.

## Complications and Considerations specific to Twin Delivery

Certain complications occur directly as a result of twin gestation. The interaction of two fetuses and their positioning and size, placement of the umbilical cords, gravida status of the mother, and method and timing of the delivery of each twin can impact the outcome of the births. Each midwife and client must work through the different scenarios possible to ensure a team effort in facilitating a good birth for each baby.

**Positioning.** Fetal positioning is one of the most important factors in planning the delivery of twin gestation. Up to 40% of all twin gestations begin labor in the vertex-vertex position, another 30% will be vertex-breech lie and 10% will be vertex-transverse (Cruikshank, 2007). The remaining 20% are in some variation of a breech first position or other presentation. At the start of labor, the midwife should be able to palpate twin A engaged in the pelvis and determine position. Ideally, twin A will be vertex. The position of twin B can be difficult to ascertain by palpation. Ultrasound confirmation of positioning near term should be considered.

Even if positioning is confirmed via ultrasound the day before labor starts, it is imperative to determine whether the babies' positioning has changed. Large fetal movements or different contours of the abdomen can indicate the need for reassessment of fetal position(s) and a change in the delivery plan (Frye, 2004). Also, 20% of second twins change position after the delivery of the first twin (Cruikshank, 2007). A midwife who intends to deliver twins at home must be prepared for all possibilities.

**Relative size of second twin compared with first twin.** In consulting with the parents and deciding on the most appropriate place of delivery, another important facet to discuss is the increased risk of fetal distress, placental separation and cord prolapse that is much more likely to occur if the second twin is 25% or more larger than the first twin (Cruikshank, 2007).

**Primipara versus multipara.** Items of concern also vary depending on number of previous births. For primiparae, the concern with a breech twin A coming through an unproven pelvis is valid. As in a singleton, primipara, breech birth, similar evaluations as to probability of success will need to be made. Although twins are usually smaller than singleton term babies, the second twin's fetal head will not have had time to mold and shape during the weeks leading up the birth, nor during a slow passage through the pelvis (Cruikshank, 2007). The same considerations need to occur in a vertex-breech presentation when twin B is substantially larger than twin A. Twin B's larger, unmolded head will need to navigate a pelvis that has only passed twin A's molded, smaller head. Both situations could theoretically cause an emergency entrapment and need to be evaluated carefully (see also Relative size of second twin vs first twin.)

For multiparae, a roomy pelvis and baggy uterus after the birth of twin A make conditions ripe for twin B to spontaneously change position, not necessarily for the better. When the mother gives birth to twin A in abdomen-dependent positions (such as hands and knees), twin B has much room to move (Frye, 2004). Utilizing gravity-dependent, upright birth positions, like squatting, standing or upright praying, can help stabilize twin B and encourage descent into the pelvis. Alternately, birth attendants can gently hold twin B externally in position after the birth of twin A until the uterus can contract around baby B. Frye (2004) suggests that, if the mom is in a standing position, the midwife, from behind the mother, reaching around the belly with her hands can palpate and guide the second twin into the mother's pelvis as the woman leans backwards into the midwife. Fundal pressure has also been suggested as a means to move the second twin into the pelvis (Fraser et al., 2003). A side-lying maternal position can stabilize baby until the mother's uterus begins contracting again and moves twin B down into position (Frye, 2004).

**Inter-twin delivery interval.** How much time to allow between the birth of each twin is a source of great debate. In the 1980's, studies touted that inter-twin delivery intervals up to 134 minutes were not associated with adverse neonatal outcomes, but recently, studies have shown a five to eight-fold increase in the need for cesarean delivery if the second twin was delivered longer than 30-60 minutes after the first twin (Cruikshank, 2007; Fraser et al., 2003). Some studies have also shown poor umbilical artery blood gas results and higher rates of cesarean delivery with longer time between twin deliveries (Lee, 2012). Schneuber and fellow researchers (2012) compared delivery intervals up to 60 minutes and found no difference in 10-minute APGAR scores nor umbilical cord pH levels (1- and 5-minute AGPAR differences were not significant) between twins with shorter inter-twin delivery time and those twin pairs with up to 60 minutes between delivery.

Chorion status can also affect planning of delivery timing of twin pairs. Although some practitioners hold the view that all monochorionic deliveries should occur by cesarean section due to the possibility of acute blood transfusion in labor, the research into the actual incidence of such transfusions does not support the practice (Devaseelan & Ong, 2010). The authors do recommend the alternative of close fetal monitoring and a short inter-twin delivery time, although they acknowledge their recommendation is without any evidence as well.

**Nuchal cords.** Unless you know that the babies are in separate sacs, it is imperative that a nuchal cord NOT be cut on the perineum. The nuchal cord could actually be from twin B and cutting it would place twin B in immediate fetal distress. Midwives must make sure to have other techniques, such as somersaulting, at their disposal as this situation could be a possibility.

**Breech first and locked twins.** Although written about quite frequently as a real, serious complication of both the breech-vertex and breech-transverse lie, one author said in 30 years of lecturing on twin deliveries, he had not encountered one provider that had experienced locked twins (Cruikshank, 2007a). He further stated that two twin studies recorded one instance each of locked twins out of, respectively, 817 and 645 twin births. Another study suggested that, although there were no locked twins in their study, there is no way of knowing how many were avoided due to planned cesarean delivery, with an additional researcher showing locked twins occurring more in primigravidas (Blickstein, Goldman, & Kupferminc, 2000; Khunda, 1972). One paper did report on instances of locked twins, one of which was resolved within 3 minutes via cesarean delivery and another where the Zavanelli maneuver was applied (Udom-Rice, Skupski, & Chervenak, 1995). Another consideration is that, even if locking does not occur (with its accompanying high fetal mortality rate), potential deflexion of the descending vertex might happen, affecting the possibility of a successful vaginal breech delivery for twin A (Udom-Rice et al., 1995).

Interlocking twins is only one type of problematic fetal positioning. Frye gives a thorough overview of how certain rare combinations of fetal positioning (collision, impaction, compaction, interlocking) can obstruct fetal descent and how to manage those situations (Frye, 2004, pp. 983-985).

Full informed consent requires a comprehensive discussion of the possible complications and must be obtained before attempting such a delivery. Still, a breech first delivery "may be safe in well defined cases" (Udom-Rice et al., 1995, p. 431).

**Version and breech extraction.** In delivering the second twin, several options are available, depending on position of the baby after the birth of twin A. If twin B is in a transverse or oblique lie, a version will be necessary to facilitate delivery. External version can be attempted, but care must be taken NOT to rupture the sac and risk trapping baby in an undeliverable position or inducing a cord prolapse. If fact, if membranes rupture before or during an internal version, risk of version failure and need for cesarean section is increased (Rebufa-Dhenin et al., 2012). A review of 118 cases of external cephalic version in second twins gave a success rate of 58% (range 46%-80%) and complications such as cord prolapse, compound presentation, fetal distress and abruption occurred in 10% of version attempts (Ramsey & Repke, 2003). "When external cephalic version is successful, amniotomy can be performed once the fetal vertex enters the pelvic inlet thus allowing the fetus to further descend into the pelvis with subsequent delivery. After a failed external cephalic version, however, the clinician must decide between an attempted operative vaginal delivery (i.e., breech extraction v internal podalic version with total breech extraction) versus cesarean delivery" (Ramsey & Repke, 2003, p. 63). If resolution to a deliverable fetal position is not possible, Frye (2004) states that transport is the safest recourse.

For babies resolving to, or in, a breech position, breech extraction has been shown to be safer than external version to a vertex position (Frye, 2004). Remember, in the midwifery model of care, the twins under discussion are term fetuses which would be larger than 1500g. All research suggests, due to fragility and the trauma that can occur during a breech delivery, that all second twins <1500g and/or extremely premature or significantly larger (25% or 500g, depending on the source) than their previously birthed twin be delivered via cesarean section for best outcomes (Cruikshank, 2007; Lee, 2012; Ramsey & Repke, 2003).

Conflicting opinions exist on using internal version in combination with breech extraction. One physician states that it should never be used, as it is "absolutely contraindicated because it is potentially dangerous and because no one trained after about 1970 has any idea how to perform the maneuver" (Cruikshank, 2007, p. 1170). In reply to these comments, Schmitz and his associates (2007) respond that they routinely do internal podalic version and subsequent breech extraction of vertex second twins to minimize inter-twin delivery times and possible need for cesarean section of the second twin. He then conveys the exact procedure they use. The procedure is given here for reference.

"As soon as the first twin is born, if the second twin fetal head is up to a 0 station, internal version is done, under peridural analgesia... The hand placed in the uterus, membranes intact, follows the back, breech, and legs of the fetus before grasping both feet. The feet are drawn down into the vagina while the external hand guides the fetal head for facilitating the rotation. The second twin is then delivered by the breech as described [in Chuikshank's article]" (Schmitz, Bernabe, Azria & Goffinet, 2007, p. 712).

They then assert that their method of delivery has resulted in a 10-20 fold decrease in the need for emergency cesareans of the second twin with no adverse neonatal outcomes. In answer, Cruikshank affirms his agreement that internal podalic version for transverse lie in the second twin is an option for those trained in the maneuver, but risks of uterine rupture, in his opinion, negate the use of the technique for delivery of a vertex twin B (Schmitz et al., 2007). In either case, if a midwife expects to use internal version along with breech extraction during a twin delivery, she should be thoroughly trained and have experience in performing the maneuver.

# 6 POSTPARTUM ISSUES IN TWIN GESTATION

Adjusting to life after a twin birth is difficult, to say the least. Physical changes, emotional outlays, and exhaustive routines quickly empty a motherly bucket that has little excess time to be filled. In looking at this process, one author dubbed it "releasing the pause button" and described four stages a mother of twins works thorough — (a) draining power, (b) pausing own life, (c) striving to reset, and (d) resuming own life, with the most taxing time being the first three months postpartum" (Beck, 2002, p. 593). Support from the midwife and the mother's social community is essential her being able to "release the pause button."

## Maternal Issues

Uterine involution will be slower in a woman after a twin birth than for a singleton mother. The extra uterine bulk takes longer to return to its original size and afterpains may be more intense as the body attempts to restore normalcy and may require analgesia. Lochia may not ease as soon due to the demands on the mother with caring for two babies. Rest should be encouraged and nutrition emphasized. Reminders from the midwife about the need for self-care as the mother cares for her new babies should be both tactful and compassionate.

Postpartum depression is more common among mothers of twins

and should be evaluated at each postpartum visit with the Edinburgh Postnatal Depression Scale (see Cox, Holden, & Sagovsky, 1987; UCSF Pediatrics, n.d.). If possible depression or suicidal thoughts are indicated, the mother needs to be referred to the appropriate healthcare providers.

## Breastfeeding

All of the normal advantages for breastfeeding newborns apply, as well as the reduced time needed for feeding once the mother can learn to tandem nurse her twins. As stated before, contact with a La Leche League leader or an International Board Certified Lactation Consultant (IBCLC) with experience supporting breastfeeding mothers of twins will be invaluable and should be initiated prenatally. The mother might be ravenous and will need a high protein, high calorie diet, eating 6-8 times per day to adequately provide nourishment for herself and to continue producing milk for her babies. Rest is also essential to producing enough milk and very hard to come by in the first weeks of life as a parent of twins. One study looked at breastfeeding twins over the first six months of life and found "that mothers who are able to persist with the difficulties of establishing a milk supply for twins and feeding two infants are able to continue providing a high percentage of the infants' feedings as breast milk" (Damato, Dowling, Madigan, & Thanattherakul, 2005, p. 201).

The midwife must walk a fine line between encouraging the breastfeeding relationship and supporting a twin mother who may not be able to adequately provide enough breastmilk to fully nourish her babies. Any breastmilk she can provide to her babies is a blessing, and the mother should be reassured of her own abilities as a parent. Otherwise, an inability to fully breastfeed for whatever reason could add to the normal stress, exhaustion and isolation of a new mother and lead to depression.

## Parental Preparation for Life After Delivery

As mentioned before, a good quality childbirth education class specifically for parents of twins will make a significant step toward healthily working through the changes in life that will occur after delivery. Discussions need to take place about the many different outcomes that can occur (possible need for hospital/NICU stays or one twin at home with another in the hospital) without creating a sense of fear or inevitability. Education on the development of twins in the first year of life, with emphasis on individuality, can be helpful as well as talking with other twin parents about family issues and dynamics, such as sibling adjustment.

Community support and outside help is critical for families adjusting to life with twin children. Twin births are associated with long term parental divorce, especially among mothers who did not complete college or who have other children already at home (Jena, Goldman, & Joyce, 2011). Fatigue, isolation and stress all contribute to parental relationship strain. It is interesting to note that one study showed fathers of twins had less sleep (almost an hour less) at two weeks after the twins were at the home than mothers, although neither averaged more than 6.5 hours of sleep (Damato & Burant, 2008). Midwives should be cognizant of the needs of the entire family as the adjustment process occurs postpartum.

Some families and communities have made volunteer schedules in four hour blocks to come and help with older childcare, dinners, laundry, household cleaning, and other chores. Help with the babies should be given at the mother's request, though. Some mothers are very open to help with their newborns whereas other mothers would like the time to bond and just be able to focus their energy on developing a relationship with each of the new babies. Sensitivity and open communication can help the midwife and community assess the needs of the new parents and offer appropriate help.

# 7 IMPORTANCE OF PROFESSIONAL RELATIONSHIPS

Midwives belong to many different communities. They have their neighborhood, their church family, possible civic groups and other circles with whom they associate. Each group has different rules, both written and unwritten, that affect the workings of that specific community. In their professional lives, they connect with many other types of health care workers, such as doulas, apprentices/student midwives, nurses, ultrasound techs, laboratory specialists, obstetricians, maternal-fetal medicine specialists and other midwives. The maternity care community, like other groups, has similar written and unwritten rules for practice and participation. These will vary by regional location (both metropolitan areas [unwritten] and state governing bodies [written]), professional guilds (possible written or unwritten), and personal practice groups.

## Standards of Practice

Delivering twins in homes and birth centers is currently a matter of great controversy. Although 1/3 of CPMs believe twins are within their scope of practice, their ability to manage such pregnancies is variable (Darragh, 2012). Some jurisdictions have made midwife-managed twins in homes and birth centers completely illegal and under the purview of obstetricians. In other places midwifery management is legal, but unwritten community standards make midwives question the wisdom in managing such pregnancies, whether or not such questioning is justified.

Still different communities allow for midwife-led home and birth center twin management within certain guidelines, such as Oregon, which allows certain twin management after consultation another licensed health-care provider except in cases of mono-mono twins, TTTS or a transverse presenting first twin; Texas, which requires the midwife to refer a multiple gestation client to physician care, and such a referral can be refused with the midwife continuing to provide care for the multiple gestation; or Manitoba, which allows both breech and twin home delivery when recommended by an obstetrician (College of Midwives of Manitoba, 2007; Oregon Board of Direct Entry Midwifery, 2011; Texas Midwifery Board, 2014).

When a midwife decides to include twins within her personal scope of practice, she must be sure that such a decision is in the best interests of both her clients and their babies and the community as well. Quality access to consultation with other providers and good protocols for transfers of care, when necessary, should be established before enrolling a mother expecting twins in care. Practice guidelines and some absolute protocols should be determined before a situation arises, so boundaries and decision-making are not made during an emotionally charged crisis. Experience under the tutelage of a midwife who has managed care for many twin mothers is invaluable before including twins within a personal scope of practice, but such opportunities are becoming increasingly rare as the legality of managing twins in homes and birth centers is being removed.

## MANA Statistics Project

Evidence-based health care has been defined as "using the best research about the safety and effectiveness of specific interventions to help guide clinical decision-making" (Sakala & Corry, 2001, p. 127). In writing this management guide, the paucity of current evidence for twin management from a midwifery background was astounding. Since relegating twins to the "high-risk" category, modern obstetrics has all but stopped doing twin research from a "normal until proven otherwise" perspective. Further, research on twins in settings where physiologic birth is facilitated is deeply lacking. Thus, if you are a midwife that manages and delivers twins in home and birth center settings, please consider submitting your data to the MANA Statistics Project database (www.manastats.org). With data, more research can be done to inform both good midwifery practices and better understanding of the "not normal" aspects of twins, so all babies can have the best start possible.

# 8 CONCLUSION

It is a well-established fact that planned home birth with a trained attendant gives positive results and allows for "high rates of physiologic birth and low rates of intervention without an increase in adverse outcomes" (Cheyney et al., 2014, p. 17; see also Hutton, Reitsma, & Kaufman, 2009; Lindgren, Radestad, Christensson, & Hildingsson, 2008; Symon, Winter, Inkster, & Donnan, 2009). Although ACOG specified twin birth as having a greater risk of perinatal death and asserted that twin gestation places a candidate at too high a risk for home birth, "there are no national guidelines in the United States that list conditions for which home birth is not recommended" (ACOG Committee on Obstetric Practice, 2011; Likis, 2014, p. 567). Despite lack of consensus and clarity in guidelines, midwives continue to facilitate home and birth center births with mothers having a twin gestation.

However, as more twin gestations become automatically escalated in care to specialists for maternity care and delivery, the "loss of core childbearing knowledge and skills among health professionals" for managing twin gestation and twin vaginal delivery seems inevitable (Sakala & Corry, 2008, p. 5). Preservation of such knowledge and skills is essential; the steep learning curve of rediscovery, should it be required, may lead to unnecessary morbidity and mortality outcomes as skill sets are re-learned and incorporated into standard of care training and scopes of practice. Examination of the current evidence led Hofmeyr, Barrett and Crowther (2011) to conclude "there is a lack of robust evidence to guide clinical advice regarding the method of birth for twin pregnancies" (p. 2). Indeed, defaulting to cesarean section in twin gestation brings with it both complications inherent to surgical procedures as well as limits to future reproductive choices for women.

While midwives "value and have a preference for normal birth,

> …we acknowledge that each birth is an individual journey and there are times when intervention is appropriate. Indeed, midwives need to do everything in their power to support and enhance the woman's positive sense of self and connection with her unborn and newborn baby, regardless of how the pregnancy, labour and birth progresses" (Fahy, Fouler & Hastie, 2008, p. ix).

By reclaiming twin birth, midwives will recover guardianship of normalcy within a birth territory that has been all but completely moved to the obstetric paradigm. It is hoped that this text may serve as a beginning point in helping midwives acquire that clinical knowledge and skill set needed to successfully guide appropriate twin gestation within a home and birth center scope of practice. As more data is made available, through resources such as the MANA Statistics Database, best practices can be found to better inform midwifery twin management.

# APPENDIX A

## Prenatal Visit Plan for Twins

Visits monthly, every 2 weeks starting at 14 weeks, weekly from 32 weeks

Midwife should allow more time for each visit when compared to a singleton mom

Discuss:

- Diet and Nutrition
- Preterm Labor S/S
- Pyelonephritis S/S
- SROM S/S
- PIH S/S
- Placental Abruption S/S
- Any lab or ultrasound results
- Appropriate discussion checklist items

Evaluate:

- Weight Gain
- Blood Pressure
- Fundal and Girth Measurements
- Fetal Heart Tones (at least ten beats per minute difference to assure two different babies)

Labs

Plan for next appointment

# APPENDIX B

## WAPF Diet for Pregnant and Nursing Mothers[1]

Daily Requirement Intake:

- Cod Liver Oil to supply 20,000 IU vitamin A and 2000 IU vitamin D per day
- 1 quart (or 32 ounces) whole milk daily, preferably raw and from pasture-fed cows (learn more about raw milk on our website, A Campaign for Real Milk, www.realmilk.com)
- 4 tablespoons butter daily, preferably from pasture-fed cows
- 2 or more eggs daily, preferably from pastured chickens
- Additional egg yolks daily, added to smoothies, salad dressings, scrambled eggs, etc.
- 3-4 ounces fresh liver, once or twice per week (If you have been told to avoid liver for fear of getting "too much Vitamin A," be sure to read Vitamin A Saga)
- Fresh seafood, 2-4 times per week, particularly wild salmon, shellfish and fish eggs
- Fresh beef or lamb daily, always consumed with the fat
- Oily fish or lard daily, for vitamin D
- 2 tablespoons coconut oil daily, used in cooking or smoothies, etc.
- Lacto-fermented condiments and beverages
- Bone broths used in soups, stews and sauces
- Soaked whole grains
- Fresh vegetables and fruits

AVOID:

- Trans fatty acids (e.g., hydrogenated oils)
- Junk foods

---

[1] Taken from Weston A. Price Foundation (WAPF). (2004). *Diet for pregnant and nursing mothers*. Retrieved February 1, 2014, from http://www.westonaprice.org/childrens-health/diet-for-pregnant-and-nursing-mothers. Copyright © 2004 by Weston A. Price Foundation. Reprinted with permission.

- Commercial fried foods
- Sugar
- White flour
- Soft drinks
- Caffeine
- Alcohol
- Cigarettes
- Drugs (even prescription drugs)

**IMPORTANT WARNING:** Cod liver oil contains substantial levels of omega-3 EPA, which can cause numerous health problems, such as hemorrhaging during the birth process, if not balanced by arachidonic acid (ARA), an omega-6 fatty acid found in liver, egg yolks and meat fats. Please do not add cod liver oil to a diet that is deficient in these important animal foods. It is important to follow our diet for pregnant mothers in its entirety, not just selected parts of it.

# APPENDIX C

## Discussion checklist additions/changes

**10-13 weeks**

Ultrasound (or as early as possible if later to care) to determine chorionicity

**14 weeks**

Discuss twin childbirth education classes

**16-24 weeks**

Ultrasound every 2 weeks to check for TTTS in MC pregnancies

**16 weeks**

Followup on twin class registration

**20 weeks**

Consider requiring anatomy ultrasound for all twin mothers due to higher rates of abnormalities

Hgb check (in addition to the normal Hgb check at 28 weeks)

**24 weeks**

Car seat reminder

Connection with twin groups in community

Discuss postpartum plans and need to begin making arrangements

**28 weeks**

Begin discussion on delivery outcomes

Infant feeding plan/connection with breastfeeding specialist

**32-36 weeks**

Consider covering all 37+ week topics by 36 weeks

Newborn issues (vitamin K, hearing screen, etc)

Home visit

Pediatrician selection, etc

# APPENDIX D

## The Art of Twin Birth

Bell, L. (n.d.). *A Babies Story: I Had a Twin Home Birth.* Retrieved from http://twiniversity.com/2014/04/a-babies-story-i-had-a-twin-home-birth/.

Bring Birth Home. (2010). *Ezra and Jude: Twin Home birth Story.* Retrieved from http://bringbirthhome.com/birth-at-home/home-birth-stories/ezra-and-jude-twin-home-birth-story/

Caines, J. (2006). *Majella and Rose's Twin Home Water Birth.* Retrieved from http://www.homebirth.org.uk/justine.htm

Gaskin, I. M. (2002). Twin Birthing on the Farm from *Spiritual midwifery* (4th ed.). Summertown, Tenn.: Book Pub. Co., 130-132.

Gentle Beginnings Homebirth Midwifery. (2015). *Kathy's Story - Full Term Twins.* Retrieved from http://homebirthbaby.net/birth-stories/kathys-story-full-term-twins/

Jemleland, J. (2008). A Father's Birth Story of Breech Twins: Tiernan Shae and Caulla Anora Mae. *Midwifery Today, 86,* 12-13, 65-66.

Nebraska Friends of Midwives. (n.d.). *Liam and Noah- Nebraska Home Birth of twins with a Non-Nurse Midwife.* Retrieved from http://nefriendsofmidwives.weebly.com/melissa--twins-home-birth.html

Nicholson, S. (2013). *Twin Home Birth.* Retrieved from https://www.youtube.com/watch?v=oCsjBZiDc6Y

Tully. G. (2013). First Twin: Breech. *Midwifery Today, 106,* 9-11.

# REFERENCES

Aaronson, D., Harlev, A., Sheiner, E., & Levy, A. (2010). Trial of labor after cesarean section in twin pregnancies: maternal and neonatal safety. *Journal of Maternal-Fetal and Neonatal Medicine, 23*(6), 550-554. doi: 10.3109/14767050903156700

ACOG Committee on Obstetric Practice. (2011). ACOG Committee Opinion No. 476: Planned home birth. *Obstetrics and Gynecology, 117*(2 Pt 1), 425-428.

Adamowicz, R., Przybylkowska, M., Trzeciak-Supel, E., & Filipp, E. (2004). [Case report of 18 weeks delayed delivery of the second twin after the miscarriage of the first fetus at the 17th week of pregnancy]. *Ginekologia Polska, 75*(1), 53-57.

Albers, L. L., & Katz, V. L. (1991). Birth setting for low-risk pregnancies: An analysis of the current literature. *Journal of Nurse-Midwifery, 36*(4), 215-220.

Al-Kuran, O., Al-Mehaisen, L., Bawadi, H., Beitawi, S., & Amarin, Z. (2011). The effect of late pregnancy consumption of date fruit on labour and delivery. *Journal of Obstetrics and Gynaecology, 31*(1), 29-31. doi: 10.3109/01443615.2010.522267

Allen, V. M., Wilson, R. D., Cheung, A., Genetics Committee of the Society of Obstetricians & Gynaecologists of Canada, & Reproductive Endocrinology Infertility Committee of the Society of Obstetricians Gynaecologists of Canada. (2006). Pregnancy outcomes after assisted reproductive technology. *Journal of Obstetrics and Gynaecology of Canada, 28*(3), 220-250.

Allison, J. (1996). *Delivered at Home.* London: Chapman & Hall.

American College of Nurse-Midwives (ACNM). (2010). Intermittent auscultation for intrapartum fetal heart rate surveillance. *Journal of Midwifery & Women's Health, 55*(4), 397-403. doi: 10.1016/j.jmwh.2010.05.007

American College of Obstetricians and Gynecologists (ACOG) Committee on Practice Bulletins-Obstetrics. (2012). ACOG practice bulletin no. 127: Management of preterm labor. *Obstetrics & Gynecology, 119*(6), 1308-1317. doi: 10.1097/AOG.0b013e31825af2f0

American College of Obstetricians & Gynecologists (ACOG), Society for Maternal-Fetal Medicine, Caughey, A. B., Cahill, A. G., Guise, J. M., & Rouse, D. J. (2014). Safe prevention of the primary cesarean delivery.

*American Journal of Obstetrics & Gynecology, 210*(3), 179-193. doi: 10.1016/j.ajog.2014.01.026

Anderson, B. A., & Stone, S. E. (2013). *Best practices in midwifery : using the evidence to implement change.* New York: Springer.

Anderson, R. E., & Murphy, P. A. (1995). Outcomes of 11,788 planned home births attended by certified nurse-midwives. A retrospective descriptive study. *Journal of Nurse-Midwifery, 40*(6), 483-492.

Ballard, C. K., Bricker, L., Reed, K., Wood, L., & Neilson, J. P. (2011). Nutritional advice for improving outcomes in multiple pregnancies. *Cochrane Database of Systematic Reviews*(6), CD008867. doi: 10.1002/14651858.CD008867.pub2

Barrett, J., & Bocking, A. (2000). Management of twin pregnancies (part 1). Retrieved November 9, 2013, from http://sogc.org/wp-content/uploads/2013/01/91E-CONS1-July2000.pdf

Bastian, H., Keirse, M. J., & Lancaster, P. A. (1998). Perinatal death associated with planned home birth in Australia: population based study. *BMJ, 317*(7155), 384-388.

Beck, C. T. (2002). Releasing the pause button: mothering twins during the first year of life. *Qualitative Health Research, 12*(5), 593-608.

Blickstein, I., Goldman, R. D., & Kupferminc, M. (2000). Delivery of breech first twins: a multicenter retrospective study. *Obstetrics & Gynecology, 95*(1), 37-42.

Blickstein, I., & Perlman, S. (2013). Single fetal death in twin gestations. *Journal of Perinatal Medicine, 41*(1). doi: 10.1515/jpm-2012-0019

Borzychowski, A. M., Sargent, I. L., & Redman, C. W. (2006). Inflammation and preeclampsia. *Seminars in Fetal and Neonatal Medicine, 11*(5), 309-316. doi: 10.1016/j.siny.2006.04.001

Boulet, S. L., Schieve, L. A., Nannini, A., Ferre, C., Devine, O., Cohen, B., . . . Macaluso, M. (2008). Perinatal outcomes of twin births conceived using assisted reproduction technology: a population-based study. *Human Reproduction, 23*(8), 1941-1948. doi: 10.1093/humrep/den169

Brent, R. L., Hendrickx, A. G., Holmes, L. B., & Miller, R. K. (1996). Teratogenicity of high vitamin A intake. *New England Journal of Medicine, 334*(18), 1196; author reply 1197.

Brewer Diet. (2005). Retrieved February 1, 2014, from http://www.preeclampsia.org/forum/viewtopic.php?t=9742

Brewer, T. (2013). Brewer diet for healthy pregnancy. Retrieved February 1, 2014, from http://blueribbonbaby.org/healthy-pregnancy/brewer-diet-for-healthy-pregnancy/

Brubaker, S. G., & Gyamfi, C. (2012). Prediction and prevention of spontaneous preterm birth in twin gestations. *Seminars in Perinatology, 36*(3), 190-194. doi: 10.1053/j.semperi.2012.02.003

Buhling, K. J., Henrich, W., Starr, E., Lubke, M., Bertram, S., Siebert, G., & Dudenhausen, J. W. (2003). Risk for gestational diabetes and hypertension for women with twin pregnancy compared to singleton pregnancy. *Archives of Gynecology and Obstetrics, 269*(1), 33-36. doi: 10.1007/s00404-003-0483-z

Challem, J. J. (1996). Teratogenicity of high vitamin A intake. *New England Journal of Medicine, 334*(18), 1196-1197.

Cheng, Y. W., Snowden, J. M., King, T. L., & Caughey, A. B. (2013). Selected perinatal outcomes associated with planned home births in the United States. *American Journal of Obstetrics & Gynecology, 209*(4), 325 e321-328. doi: 10.1016/j.ajog.2013.06.022

Cheyney, M., Bovbjerg, M., Everson, C., Gordon, W., Hannibal, D., & Vedam, S. (2014). Outcomes of care for 16,924 planned home births in the United States: the midwives alliance of north america statistics project, 2004 to 2009. *Journal of Midwifery & Women's Health, 59*(1), 17-27. doi:10.1111/jmwh.12172

College of Midwives of Manitoba. (2007). *Standard for Discussion, Consultation and Transfer of Care*. Retrieved from http://www.midwives.mb.ca/policies_and_standards/standard-discussion-consultation-and-transfer-of-care.pdf

Cook, E., Avery, M., & Frisvold, M. (2014). Formulating evidence-based guidelines for certified nurse-midwives and certified midwives attending home births. *Journal of Midwifery & Women's Health, 59*(2), 153-159. doi: 10.1111/jmwh.12142

Cox, J. L., Holden, J. M., & Sagovsky, R. (1987). Detection of postnatal depression. Development of the 10-item Edinburgh Postnatal Depression Scale. *British Journal of Psychiatry, 150*, 782-786.

Cruikshank, D. P. (2007). Intrapartum management of twin gestations. *Obstetrics & Gynecology, 109*(5), 1167-1176. doi: 10.1097/01.AOG.0000260387.69720.5d

Cruz, M., Foeller, M., Zhao, S., & Szabo, A. (2014). Are adverse neonate outcomes in gestational diabetes mellitus twin gestations decreased compared with nondiabetic twins? *Obstetrics & Gynecology, 123* Suppl 1, 46S. doi: 10.1097/01.AOG.0000447330.83496.38

D'Antonio, F., Khalil, A., Dias, T., Thilaganathan, B., & Southwest Thames Obstetric Research. (2013). Early fetal loss in monochorionic and dichorionic twin pregnancies: analysis of the Southwest Thames Obstetric Research Collaborative (STORK) multiple pregnancy cohort. *Ultrasound in Obstetrics and Gynecology, 41*(6), 632-636. doi: 10.1002/uog. 12363

Damato, E. G., & Burant, C. (2008). Sleep patterns and fatigue in parents of twins. *Journal of Obstetric, Gynecologic, and Neonatal Nursing, 37*(6), 738-749. doi: 10.1111/j.1552-6909.2008.00296.x

Damato, E. G., Dowling, D. A., Madigan, E. A., & Thanattherakul, C. (2005). Duration of breastfeeding for mothers of twins. *Journal of Obstetric, Gynecologic, and Neonatal Nursing, 34*(2), 201-209. doi: 10.1177/0884217504273671

Darragh, I. (2012). Certified professional midwives: Where are they? What are they doing? Where are the challenges in licensure and scope of practice? *CPM Symposium.* Warrenton, Virginia.

Devaseelan, P., & Ong, S. (2010). Twin pregnancy: controversies in management. *The Obstetrician & Gynaecologist, 12*(3), 179-185. doi: 10.1576/toag.12.3.179.27600

Devoe, L. D. (2008). Antenatal fetal assessment: multifetal gestation--an overview. *Seminars in Perinatology, 32*(4), 281-287. doi: 10.1053/ j.semperi.2008.04.011

Edmonds, K. (2007). *Dewhurst's textbook of obstetrics and gynaecology (7th ed.).* Malden, Massachusetts: Blackwell Publishing.

Eleje, G. U., Ofojebe, C. J., Udegbunam, O. I., & Adichie, C. V. (2014). Determinants of umbilical cord prolapse in a low-resource setting. *Journal of Women's Health, Issues & Care, 3*(1), 1-4. doi: 10.4172/2325-9795.1000132

Fahy, K., Foureur, M., & Hastie, C. (2008). *Birth territory and midwifery guardianship: theory for practice, education, and research.* Edinburgh: New York: Books for Midwives.

Fraser, D., Cooper, M. A., & Myles, M. F. (2003). *Myles textbook for midwives (14th ed.).* Edinburgh ; New York: Churchill Livingstone.

Fraser, D., Cooper, M. A., & Myles, M. F. (2009). *Myles textbook for midwives (15th ed.).* Edinburgh ; New York: Churchill Livingstone.

Frezza, S., Gallini, F., Puopolo, M., De Carolis, M. P., D'Andrea, V., Guidone, P. I., . . . Romagnoli, C. (2011). Is growth-discordance in twins a substantial risk factor in adverse neonatal outcomes? *Twin Research and Human Genetics, 14*(5), 463-467. doi: 10.1375/twin.14.5.463

Frye, A. (2004). *Holistic midwifery : A comprehensive textbook for midwives in homebirth practice (1st ed. Vol. 2).* Portland, OR: Labrys Press.

Frye, A. (2010). *Healing passage: A midwife's guide to the care and repair of the tissues involved in birth (6th ed.)*. Portland, OR: Labrys Press.

Gabbe, S. G., Niebyl, J. R., & Simpson, J. L. (2007). *Obstetrics: normal and problem pregnancies (5th ed.)*. Philadelphia, PA: Churchill Livingstone/ Elsevier.

Gavard, J. A., & Artal, R. (2014). Gestational weight gain and maternal and neonatal outcomes in term twin pregnancies in obese women. *Twin Research and Human Genetics, 17*(2), 127-133. doi: 10.1017/thg.2013.91

Ghomian, N., Hafizi, L., & Takhti, Z. (2013). The role of vitamin C in prevention of preterm premature rupture of membranes. *Iranian Red Crescent Medical Journal, 15*(2), 113-116. doi: 10.5812/ircmj.5138

Gibbs, R. S., Romero, R., Hillier, S. L., Eschenbach, D. A., & Sweet, R. L. (1992). A review of premature birth and subclinical infection. *American Journal of Obstetrics & Gynecology, 166*(5), 1515-1528.

Glinianaia, S. V., Rankin, J., & Wright, C. (2008). Congenital anomalies in twins: a register-based study. *Human Reproduction, 23*(6), 1306-1311. doi: 10.1093/humrep/den104

Gratacos, E., Ortiz, J. U., & Martinez, J. M. (2012). A systematic approach to the differential diagnosis and management of the complications of monochorionic twin pregnancies. *Fetal Diagnosis and Therapy, 32*(3), 145-155. doi: 10.1159/000342751

Grünebaum, A., McCullough, L. B., Brent, R. L., Arabin, B., Levene, M. I., & Chervenak, F. A. (2015). Perinatal risks of planned home births in the United States. *American Journal of Obstetrics & Gynecology, 212*(3), 350 e351-356. doi: 10.1016/j.ajog.2014.10.021

Guillen, M. A., Herranz, L., Barquiel, B., Hillman, N., Burgos, M. A., & Pallardo, L. F. (2014). Influence of gestational diabetes mellitus on neonatal weight outcome in twin pregnancies. *Diabetic Medicine, 31*(12), 1651-1656. doi: 10.1111/dme.12523

Henry, D. E., McElrath, T. F., & Smith, N. A. (2013). Preterm severe preeclampsia in singleton and twin pregnancies. *Journal of Perinatology, 33*(2), 94-97. doi: 10.1038/jp.2012.74

Herrera, B. (2012). Brewer diet be damned. Retrieved February 1, 2014, from http://navelgazingmidwife.squarespace.com/navelgazing-midwife-blog/2012/10/20/brewer-diet-be-damned.html

Hillman, S. C., Morris, R. K., & Kilby, M. D. (2011). Co-twin prognosis after single fetal death: a systematic review and meta-analysis. *Obstetrics & Gynecology, 118*(4), 928-940. doi: 10.1097/AOG.0b013e31822f129d

Hofmeyr, G. J., Barrett, J. F. & Crowther, C. A. (2011). Planned cesarean section for women with a twin pregnancy. *Cochrane Database of Systematic Reviews*(12), CD006553. doi: 10.1002/14651858.CD006553.pub2

Hutton, E. K., Reitsma, A. H., & Kaufman, K. (2009). Outcomes associated with planned home and planned hospital births in low-risk women attended by midwives in Ontario, Canada, 2003-2006: a retrospective cohort study. *Birth, 36*(3), 180-189. doi: 10.1111/j.1523-536X.2009.00322.x

Janssen, P. A., Lee, S. K., Ryan, E. M., Etches, D. J., Farquharson, D. F., Peacock, D., & Klein, M. C. (2002). Outcomes of planned home births versus planned hospital births after regulation of midwifery in British Columbia. *Canadian Medical Association Journal, 166*(3), 315-323.

Jena, A. B., Goldman, D. P., & Joyce, G. (2011). Association between the birth of twins and parental divorce. *Obstetrics & Gynecology, 117*(4), 892-897. doi: 10.1097/AOG.0b013e3182102adf

Johnson, C. D., & Zhang, J. (2002). Survival of other fetuses after a fetal death in twin or triplet pregnancies. *Obstetrics & Gynecology, 99*(5 Pt 1), 698-703.

Johnson, K. C., & Daviss, B. A. (2005). Outcomes of planned home births with certified professional midwives: large prospective study in North America. *BMJ, 330*(7505), 1416.

Kato, N., & Matsuda, T. (2006). Estimation of optimal birth weights and gestational ages for twin births in Japan. *BMC Public Health*, 6, 45. doi: 10.1186/1471-2458-6-45

Kennare, R. M., Keirse, M. J., Tucker, G. R., & Chan, A. C. (2010). Planned home and hospital births in South Australia, 1991-2006: differences in outcomes. *Medical Journal of Australia, 192*(2), 76-80. doi: ken10465_fm

Khadem, N., Sharaphy, A., Latifnejad, R., Hammod, N., & Ibrahimzadeh, S. (2007). Comparing the Efficacy of Dates and Oxytocin in the Management of Postpartum Hemorrhage. *Shiraz E-Medical Journal, 8*(2), 64-71.

Khunda, S. (1972). Locked twins. *Obstetrics & Gynecology, 39*(3), 453-459.

Klein, K., Mailath-Pokorny, M., Leipold, H., Krampl-Bettelheim, E., & Worda, C. (2010). Influence of gestational diabetes mellitus on weight discrepancy in twin pregnancies. *Twin Research and Human Genetics, 13*(4), 393-397. doi: 10.1375/twin.13.4.393

Lannon, S. M., Vanderhoeven, J. P., Eschenbach, D. A., Gravett, M. G., & Adams Waldorf, K. M. (2014). Synergy and interactions among biological pathways leading to preterm premature rupture of membranes. *Reproductive Sciences, 21*(10), 1215-1227. doi: 10.1177/1933719114534535

Lato, K., Berg, C., Gembruch, U., & Geipel, A. (2009). Prenatal diagnosis of structural abnormalities in monochorionic and dichorionic twin pregnancies. Paper presented at the *19th World Congress on Ultrasound in Obstetrics and Gynecology,* Hamburg, Germany.

Lay, M. M. (2000). *The rhetoric of midwifery : gender, knowledge, and power.* New Brunswick, N.J.: Rutgers University Press.

Lee, H., Wagner, A. J., Sy, E., Ball, R., Feldstein, V. A., Goldstein, R. B., & Farmer, D. L. (2007). Efficacy of radiofrequency ablation for twin-reversed arterial perfusion sequence. *American Journal of Obstetrics & Gynecology, 196*(5), 459 e451-454. doi: 10.1016/j.ajog.2006.11.039

Lee, Y. M. (2012). Delivery of twins. *Seminars in Perinatology, 36*(3), 195-200. doi: 10.1053/j.semperi.2012.02.004

Lee, Y. M., Cleary-Goldman, J., & D'Alton, M. E. (2006). Multiple gestations and late preterm (near-term) deliveries. *Seminars in Perinatology, 30*(2), 103-112. doi: 10.1053/j.semperi. 2006.03.001

Leftwich, H. K., Zaki, M. N., Wilkins, I., & Hibbard, J. U. (2013). Labor patterns in twin gestations. *American Journal of Obstetrics & Gynecology, 209*(3), 254 e251-255. doi: 10.1016/j.ajog.2013.06.019

Leveno, K. J., & Alexander, J. M. (2013). *Williams manual of pregnancy complications (23rd ed.).* New York: McGraw-Hill Professional.

Li, Y., Townend, J., Rowe, R., Brocklehurst, P., Knight, M., Linsell, L., . . . Hollowell, J. (2015). Perinatal and maternal outcomes in planned home and obstetric unit births in women at 'higher risk' of complications: secondary analysis of the Birthplace national prospective cohort study. *BJOG, 122*(5), 741-753. doi: 10.1111/1471-0528.13283

Likis, F. E. (2011). Midwives are essential to global maternal and child health. *Journal of Midwifery & Women's Health, 56*(5), 425-426. doi: 10.1111/j.1542-2011.2011.00114.x

Lin, M. G. (2006). Umbilical cord prolapse. *Obstetrical and Gynecological Survey, 61*(4), 269-277. doi: 10.1097/01.ogx.0000208802.20908.c6

Lindgren, H. E., Radestad, I. J., Christensson, K., & Hildingsson, I. M. (2008). Outcome of planned home births compared to hospital births in Sweden between 1992 and 2004. A population-based register study. *Acta Obstetricia et Gynecologica Scandinavica, 87*(7), 751-759. doi: 10.1080/00016340802199903

Linskens, I. H., Elburg, R. M., Oepkes, D., Vugt, J. M., & Haak, M. C. (2011). Expectant management in twin pregnancies with discordant structural fetal anomalies. *Twin Research and Human Genetics, 14*(3), 283-289. doi: 10.1375/twin.14.3.283

Luke, B. (2005a). Nutrition in multiple gestations. *Clinics in Perinatology, 32*(2), 403-429, vii. doi: 10.1016/j.clp.2005.02.005

Luke, B. (2005b). Nutrition and multiple gestation. *Seminars in Perinatology, 29*(5), 349-354. doi: 10.1053/j.semperi.2005.08.004

Luke, B., Brown, M. B., Misiunas, R., Anderson, E., Nugent, C., van de Ven, C., . . . Gogliotti, S. (2003). Specialized prenatal care and maternal and infant outcomes in twin pregnancy. *American Journal of Obstetrics & Gynecology, 189*(4), 934-938.

Luke, B., Brown, M. B., Nugent, C., Gonzalez-Quintero, V. H., Witter, F. R., & Newman, R. B. (2004). Risk factors for adverse outcomes in spontaneous versus assisted conception twin pregnancies. *Fertility and Sterility, 81*(2), 315-319. doi: 10.1016/j.fertnstert.2003.07.012

Luke, B., & Eberlein, T. (2011). *When you're expecting twins, triplets, or quads: Proven guidelines for a healthy multiple pregnancy (3rd ed.).* New York: Harper.

MacDorman, M. F., Declercq, E., & Mathews, T. J. (2013). Recent trends in out-of-hospital births in the United States. *Journal of Midwifery & Women's Health, 58*(5), 494-501. doi: 10.1111/jmwh.12092

Madrona, M., & Mehl-Madrona, L. (1998). Letters to the Editor. *Journal of Nurse-Midwifery, 43*(2), 2.

Major, H. D., Campbell, R. A., Silver, R. M., Branch, D. W., & Weyrich, A. S. (2014). Synthesis of sFlt-1 by platelet-monocyte aggregates contributes to the pathogenesis of preeclampsia. *American Journal of Obstetrics & Gynecology, 210*(6), 547.e1-7. doi:10.1016/j.ajog.2014.01.024

Margulis, J. (2013). Are ultrasounds causing autism in unborn babies? *Pathways to Family Wellness*(40), 46-49.

Mehl, L. E., Ramiel, J. R., Leininger, B., Hoff, B., Kronenthal, K., & Peterson, G. H. (1980). Evaluation of outcomes of non-nurse midwives: matched comparisons with physicians. *Women & Health, 5*(2), 17-29.

Mehl-Madrona, L., & Madrona, M. M. (1997). Physician- and midwife-attended home births. Effects of breech, twin, and post-dates outcome data on mortality rates. *Journal of Nurse-Midwifery, 42*(2), 91-98.

Metzger, B. E., Buchanan, T. A., Coustan, D. R., de Leiva, A., Dunger, D. B., Hadden, D. R., . . . Zoupas, C. (2007). Summary and recommendations of the Fifth International Workshop-Conference on Gestational Diabetes Mellitus. *Diabetes Care, 30* Suppl 2, S251-260. doi: 10.2337/

dc07-s225

Midwifery Task Force. (2008). *The Midwives Model of Care.* Retrieved February 1, 2014, from http://cfmidwifery.org/mmoc/define.aspx

Midwifery Today. (2013). *Midwifery today, issue 110, summer 2013.* Retrieved from http://www.midwiferytoday.com/magazine/issue110.asp

Miller, J., Chauhan, S. P., & Abuhamad, A. Z. (2012). Discordant twins: diagnosis, evaluation and management. *American Journal of Obstetrics & Gynecology, 206*(1), 10-20. doi: 10.1016/j.ajog.2011.06.075

Morikawa, M., Yamada, T., Yamada, T., Sato, S., & Minakami, H. (2012). Prospective risk of intrauterine fetal death in monoamniotic twin pregnancies. *Twin Research and Human Genetics, 15*(4), 522-526. doi: 10.1017/thg.2012.30

Morin, L., & Lim, K. (2011). Ultrasound in twin pregnancies. *Journal of Obstetrics and Gynaecology Canada, 33*(6), 643-656.

National Institute of Health and Care Excellence (NICE). (2011). Multiple pregnancy: The management of twin and triplet pregnancies in the antenatal period. Quick reference guide. In *National Collaborating Centre for Women's and Children's Health (NCC-WCH).* NICE clinical guideline 129.

National Research Council. (2009). *Weight gain during pregnancy: Reexamining the guidelines.* Washington, DC: The National Academies Press.

North American Registry of Midwives. (2014). *Shared decision making and informed consent.* Retrieved from http://narm.org/accountability/informed-consent/

Norwitz, E. R., Edusa, V., & Park, J. S. (2005). Maternal physiology and complications of multiple pregnancy. *Seminars in Perinatology, 29*(5), 338-348. doi: 10.1053/j.semperi.2005.08.002

O'Sullivan, J. V. (1968). Multiple pregnancy. *Proceedings of the Royal Society of Medicine, 61*(3), 234-236.

Odent, M. (2001). *Preeclampsia as a maternal-fetal conflict.* Retrieved February, 21, 2014, from http://www.medscape.com/viewarticle/429966_1

Odibo, A. O., Patel, K. R., Spitalnik, A., Odibo, L., & Huettner, P. (2014). Placental pathology, first-trimester biomarkers and adverse pregnancy outcomes. *Journal of Perinatology, 34*(3), 186-191. doi: 10.1038/jp. 2013.176

Okby, R., Shoham-Vardi, I., Ruslan, S., & Sheiner, E. (2013). Is induction of labor risky for twins compare to singleton pregnancies? *Journal of Maternal-Fetal and Neonatal Medicine, 26*(18), 1804-1806. doi: 10.3109/14767058.2013.804047

Olsen, O. (1997). Meta-analysis of the safety of home birth. *Birth, 24*(1), 4-13; discussion 14-16.

Olsen, S. F., Osterdal, M. L., Salvig, J. D., Weber, T., Tabor, A., & Secher, N. J. (2007). Duration of pregnancy in relation to fish oil supplementation and habitual fish intake: a randomised clinical trial with fish oil. *European Journal of Clinical Nutrition, 61*(8), 976-985. doi: 10.1038/sj.ejcn.1602609

Oregon Board of Direct Entry Midwifery. (2011). *Division 25 practice standards.* Retrieved November 29, 2014, from http://arcweb.sos.state.or.us/pages/rules/oars_300/oar_332/332_025.html

Osaikhuwuomwan, J. A., Okpere, E. E., Okonkwo, C. A., Ande, A. B., & Idogun, E. S. (2011). Plasma vitamin C levels and risk of preterm prelabour rupture of membranes. *Archives of Gynecology and Obstetrics, 284*(3), 593-597. doi: 10.1007/s00404-010-1741-5

Petousis, S., Goutzioulis, A., Margioula-Siarkou, C., Katsamagkas, T., Kalogiannidis, I., & Agorastos, T. (2012). Emergency cervical cerclage after miscarriage of the first fetus in dichorionic twin pregnancies: obstetric and neonatal outcomes of delayed delivery interval. *Archives of Gynecology and Obstetrics, 286*(3), 613-617. doi: 10.1007/s00404-012-2362-y

Ramsey, P. S., & Repke, J. T. (2003). Intrapartum management of multifetal pregnancies. *Seminars in Perinatology, 27*(1), 54-72.

Rauh-Hain, J. A., Rana, S., Tamez, H., Wang, A., Cohen, B., Cohen, A., . . . Thadhani, R. (2009). Risk for developing gestational diabetes in women with twin pregnancies. *Journal of Maternal-Fetal and Neonatal Medicine, 22*(4), 293-299. doi: 10.1080/14767050802663194

Rebufa-Dhenin, E., Flandrin, A., Reyftmann, L., Dechaud, H., Burlet, G., & Boulot, P. (2012). [Rupture of membranes in case of internal podalic version: a risk for cesarean section on the second twin]. *Gynécologie Obstétrique & Fertilité, 40*(7-8), 402-405. doi: 10.1016/j.gyobfe.2012.02.023

Regan, J. A., Chao, S., & James, L. S. (1981). Premature rupture of membranes, preterm delivery, and group B streptococcal colonization of mothers. *American Journal of Obstetrics & Gynecology, 141*(2), 184-186.

Romm, A. J. (2003). *The natural pregnancy book : herbs, nutrition, and other holistic choices.* Berkeley, Calif.: Celestial Arts.

Rooks, J. (1997). *Midwifery and childbirth in America.* Philadelphia: Temple University Press.

Rossi, A. C., & Prefumo, F. (2013). Impact of cord entanglement on perinatal outcome of monoamniotic twins: a systematic review of the literature. *Ultrasound in Obstetrics and Gynecology, 41*(2), 131-135. doi: 10.1002/uog.12345

Rothman, K. J., Moore, L. L., Singer, M. R., Nguyen, U. S., Mannino, S., & Milunsky, A. (1995). Teratogenicity of high vitamin A intake. *New England Journal of Medicine, 333*(21), 1369-1373. doi: 10.1056/NEJM199511233332101

Royal College of Obstetricians and Gynaecologists (RCOG). (2008). Management of monochorionic twin pregnancy. *Green-top Guideline*, 1-13.

Sackett, D. L., Rosenberg, W. M. C., Gray, J. A. M., Haynes, R. B., & Richardson, W. S. (1996). Evidence based medicine: what is it and what it isn't. *BMJ, 312,* 71-72.

Salihu, H. M., Aliyu, M. H., Sedjro, J. E., Nabukera, S., Oluwatade, O. J., & Alexander, G. R. (2005). Teen twin pregnancies: differences in fetal growth outcomes among blacks and whites. *American Journal of Perinatology, 22*(6), 335-339. doi: 10.1055/s-2005-871658

Sakala, C., & Corry, M. P. (2001). What is evidence-based health care? *Journal of Midwifery & Women's Health, 46*(3), 127-128.

Sakala, C., & Corry, M. P. (2008). *Evidence-based maternity care: What it is and what it can achieve.* Retrieved from http://www.milbank.org/uploads/documents/0809MaternityCare/0809MaternityCare.pdf

Santolaya, J., & Faro, R. (2012). Twins--twice more trouble? *Clinical Obstetrics and Gynecology, 55*(1), 296-306. doi: 10.1097/GRF.0b013e3182446f51

Schaaf, J. M., Hof, M. H., Mol, B. W., Abu-Hanna, A., & Ravelli, A. C. (2012). Recurrence risk of preterm birth in subsequent twin pregnancy after preterm singleton delivery. *BJOG, 119*(13), 1624-1629. doi: 10.1111/j.1471-0528.2012.03504.x

Schmitz, T., Bernabe, C., Azria, E., & Goffinet, F. (2007). Intrapartum management of twin gestations. *Obstetrics & Gynecology, 110*(3), 712; author reply 712. doi: 10.1097/01.AOG.0000280282.83266.15

Schneuber, S., Magnet, E., Haas, J., Giuliani, A., Freidl, T., Lang, U., & Bjelic-Radisic, V. (2012). Twin-to-Twin Delivery Time: Neonatal Outcome of the Second Twin. *Twin Research and Human Genetics, 14*(06), 573-579. doi: 10.1375/twin.14.6.573

Sebire, N. J., Snijders, R. J., Hughes, K., Sepulveda, W., & Nicolaides, K. H. (1997). The hidden mortality of monochorionic twin pregnancies. *British Journal of Obstetrics and Gynaecology, 104*(10), 1203-1207.

Sela, H. Y., & Simpson, L. L. (2011). Preterm premature rupture of membranes complicating twin pregnancy: management considerations. *Clinical Obstetrics and Gynecology, 54*(2), 321-329. doi: 10.1097/GRF. 0b013e318217d60d

Shumpert, M. N., Salihu, H. M., & Kirby, R. S. (2004). Impact of maternal anaemia on birth outcomes of teen twin pregnancies: a comparative analysis with mature young mothers. *Journal of Obstetrics and Gynaecology, 24*(1), 16-21. doi: 10.1080/01443610310001620224

Siega-Riz, A. M., Deierlein, A., & Stuebe, A. (2010). Implementation of the new institute of medicine gestational weight gain guidelines. *Journal of Midwifery & Women's Health, 55*(6), 512-519. doi: 10.1016/j.jmwh. 2010.04.001

Silver, R. K., Haney, E. I., Grobman, W. A., MacGregor, S. N., Casele, H. L., & Neerhof, M. G. (2000). Comparison of active phase labor between triplet, twin, and singleton gestations. *Journal of the Society for Gynecologic Investigation, 7*(5), 297-300.

Simoes, T., Queiros, A., Correia, L., Rocha, T., Dias, E., & Blickstein, I. (2011). Gestational diabetes mellitus complicating twin pregnancies. *Journal of Perinatal Medicine, 39*(4), 437-440. doi: 10.1515/JPM.2011.048

Simpson, K. R. (2010). NICHD Definitions and Classifications: Application to Electronic Fetal Monitoring Interpretation. *NCC Monograph, 3*(1).

Sperling, L., & Tabor, A. (2001). Twin pregnancy: the role of ultrasound in management. *Acta Obstetricia et Gynecologica Scandinavica, 80*, 287-299.

Star, W. L., Shannon, M. T., Lommel, L. L., & Gutierrez, Y. M. (1999). *Ambulatory obstetrics (3rd ed.)*. San Francisco: UCSF Nursing Press.

Suzuki, S., Hiraizumi, Y., & Miyake, H. (2012). Risk factors for postpartum hemorrhage requiring transfusion in cesarean deliveries for Japanese twins: comparison with those for singletons. *Archives of Gynecology and Obstetrics, 286*(6), 1363-1367. doi: 10.1007/s00404-012-2461-9

Symon, A., Winter, C., Inkster, M., & Donnan, P. T. (2009). Outcomes for births booked under an independent midwife and births in NHS maternity units: matched comparison study. *BMJ, 338*, b2060. doi: 10.1136/bmj.b2060

Tan, H., Wen, S. W., Walker, M., & Demissie, K. (2004). Missing paternal demographics: A novel indicator for identifying high risk population of adverse pregnancy outcomes. *BMC Pregnancy Childbirth, 4*(1), 21. doi: 10.1186/1471-2393-4-21

Texas Midwifery Board. (2014). *Midwifery Rules*. Retrieved from https:// www.dshs.state.tx.us/midwife/pdf/mw_rules2014.pdf

Tharpe, N., Farley, C. L., & Jordan, R. G. (2013). *Clinical practice guidelines for midwifery and women's health (4th ed.)*. Burlington, MA: Jones & Bartlett Learning.

Tita, A. T., Szychowski, J. M., Rouse, D. J., Bean, C. M., Chapman, V., Nothern, A., . . . Hauth, J. C. (2012). Higher-dose oxytocin and hemorrhage after vaginal delivery: a randomized controlled trial. *Obstetrics & Gynecology, 119*(2 Pt 1), 293-300. doi: 10.1097/AOG. 0b013e318242da74

Tiwari, P., Mishra, B. N., & Sangwan, N. S. (2014). Phytochemical and pharmacological properties of Gymnema sylvestre: an important medicinal plant. *BioMed Research International, 2014*, 830285. doi: 10.1155/2014/830285

Twin Source. (2013). *Midwives and twin deliveries: Interview with Maria Mayzel*. Retrieved from http://www.thetwinsource.com/index.php/en/ hospital-411/labor-a-delivery/129-interview-with-twin-mom-and-student-midwife-maria-mayzel

Twining, P., McHugo, J. M., & Pilling, D. W. (2007). *Textbook of fetal abnormalities*. Philadelphia, Pennsylvania: Churchill Livingstone Elsevier.

UCSF Pediatrics. *Edinburgh postnatal depression scale*. Retrieved November 29, 2014, from http://www.fresno.ucsf.edu/pediatrics/downloads/ edinburghscale.pdf

Udom-Rice, I., Skupski, D. W., & Chervenak, F. A. (1995). Intrapartum management of multiple gestation. *Seminars in Perinatology, 19*(5), 424-434.

Vandorsten, J. P., Dodson, W. C., Espeland, M. A., Grobman, W. A., Guise, J. M., Mercer, B. M., . . . Tita, A. T. (2013). NIH consensus development conference: diagnosing gestational diabetes mellitus. *NIH Consensus and State-of-the-Science Statements, 29*(1), 1-31.

van Alten, D., Eskes, M., & Treffers, P. E. (1989). Midwifery in the Netherlands. The Wormerveer study; selection, mode of delivery, perinatal mortality and infant morbidity. *British Journal of Obstetrics and Gynaecology, 96*(6), 656-662.

Varner, M. W., Leindecker, S., Spong, C. Y., Moawad, A. H., Hauth, J. C., Landon, M. B., . . . Human Development Maternal-Fetal Medicine Units, N. (2005). The Maternal-Fetal Medicine Unit cesarean registry: trial of labor with a twin gestation. *American Journal of Obstetrics & Gynecology, 193*(1), 135-140. doi: 10.1016/j.ajog.2005.03.023

Varney, H., Kriebs, J. M., & Gegor, C. L. (2004). *Varney's Midwifery (4th ed.)*. Sudbury, MA: Jones and Bartlett Publishers.

Vedam, S., Schummers, L., & Fulton, C. (2011). Home birth: an annotated

guide to the literature. 1-15. Retrieved from http://
www.bcmidwives.com/files/Home%20Birth%20Annotated%20guide
%20to%20the%20literature%20May%202011.pdf

Vedam, S., Stoll, K., Schummers, L., & Fulton, C. (2013). Home birth: an
annotated guide to the literature. 1-16. Retrieved from http://med-
fom-midwifery.sites.olt.ubc.ca/files/2014/01/
HomeBirth_AnnotatedGuideToTheLiterature.pdf.

Vink, J., Wapner, R., & D'Alton, M. E. (2012). Prenatal diagnosis in twin
gestations. *Seminars in Perinatology, 36*(3), 169-174. doi: 10.1053/
j.semperi.2012.02.008

Wagner, M. (1998). Letter to the Editor. *Journal of Nurse-Midwifery, 43*(2), 1.

Watkins, M., Moore, C., & Mulinare, J. (1996). Teratogenicity of high
vitamin A intake. *New England Journal of Medicine, 334*(18), 1196; author
reply 1197.

Watterberg, K. L., & AAP Committee on Fetus and Newborn. (2013).
Policy statement on planned home birth: upholding the best interests
of children and families. *Pediatrics, 132*(5), 924-926. doi: 10.1542/peds.
2013-2596

Weis, M. A., Harper, L. M., Roehl, K. A., Odibo, A. O., & Cahill, A. G.
(2012). Natural history of placenta previa in twins. *Obstetrics &
Gynecology, 120*(4), 753-758. doi: 10.1097/AOG.0b013e318269baac

Wen, S. W., Fung Kee Fung, K., Oppenheimer, L., Demissie, K., Yang, Q.,
& Walker, M. (2004). Neonatal morbidity in second twin according to
gestational age at birth and mode of delivery. *American Journal of
Obstetrics & Gynecology, 191*(3), 773-777. doi: 10.1016/j.ajog.2004.04.009

Wenckus, D. J., Gao, W., Kominiarek, M. A., & Wilkins, I. (2014). The
effects of labor and delivery on maternal and neonatal outcomes in
term twins: a retrospective cohort study. *BJOG, 121*(9), 1137-1144. doi:
10.1111/1471-0528.12642

Westhoff, G., Cotter, A. M., & Tolosa, J. E. (2013). Prophylactic oxytocin
for the third stage of labour to prevent postpartum haemorrhage.
*Cochrane Database of Systematic Reviews*(10), CD001808. doi:
10.1002/14651858.CD001808.pub2

Weston A. Price Foundation (WAPF). (2004). *Diet for pregnant and nursing
mothers*. Retrieved February 1, 2014, from http://
www.westonaprice.org/childrens-health/diet-for-pregnant-and-
nursing-mothers

Wetta, L. A., Szychowski, J. M., Seals, S., Mancuso, M. S., Biggio, J. R., &
Tita, A. T. (2013). Risk factors for uterine atony/postpartum

hemorrhage requiring treatment after vaginal delivery. *American Journal of Obstetrics & Gynecology, 209*(1), 51 e51-56. doi: 10.1016/j.ajog.2013.03.011

Williams, E. L., & Casanova, M. F. (2010). Potential teratogenic effects of ultrasound on corticogenesis: implications for autism. *Medical Hypotheses, 75*(1), 53-58. doi: 10.1016/j.mehy.2010.01.027

Williams, E. L., & Casanova, M. F. (2011). Above genetics: lessons from cerebral development in autism. *Translational Neuroscience, 2*(2), 106-120. doi: 10.2478/s13380-011-0016-3

Xu, H., Perez-Cuevas, R., Xiong, X., Reyes, H., Roy, C., Julien, P., . . . Innate Study Group. (2010). An international trial of antioxidants in the prevention of preeclampsia (INTAPP). *American Journal of Obstetrics & Gynecology, 202*(3), 239 e231-239 e210. doi: 10.1016/j.ajog.2010.01.050

Young, B. C., & Wylie, B. J. (2012). Effects of twin gestation on maternal morbidity. *Seminars in Perinatology, 36*(3), 162-168. doi: 10.1053/j.semperi.2012.02.007

Zhang, J., Meikle, S., Grainger, D. A., & Trumble, A. (2002). Multifetal pregnancy in older women and perinatal outcomes. *Fertility and Sterility, 78*(3), 562-568.

# ABOUT THE AUTHOR

A Virginia native, B. Maria Cranford, CPM MSM, is currently licensed midwife and owner of Mountain Home Birth & Midwifery, LLC in the Salt Lake area of Utah and president of the Utah Midwives Organization. Having completed her Master's of Midwifery at Midwives College of Utah and undergraduate at Brigham Young University, Maria's clinical midwifery training spanned several east coast states as well as her new home in Utah. Prior to becoming a very busy mother of 8 (soon to be 9) children, Maria enjoyed hiking, camping and curling up with a good book during a rolling thunderstorm.

www.ingramcontent.com/pod-product-compliance
Lightning Source LLC
Chambersburg PA
CBHW041932220326
41598CB00055BA/33